Writing for Health Professionals

About the Author

Philip Burnard is a Reader at the University of Wales College of Medicine, Cardiff. He is the author or editor of 30 books and more than 200 papers in journals and magazines. His work has been published in the UK, USA, Italy, Czech Republic, Finland and Hong Kong and has been translated into various languages. He is a book, computer software and manuscript reviewer for a range of journals, on the editorial boards of four international journals and an editorial adviser to various publishing companies. He is also the editor of a series of research monographs.

Dr Burnard has carried out research into counselling, interpersonal communication, experiential learning, reflective practice, forensic psychiatry and attitudes towards mental health. He is an honorary lecturer at the Hogeschool Midden Nederland, Utrecht, Netherlands and a visiting lecturer at universities and colleges in Sweden, Hong Kong, Finland, Brunei and Curacao. He lives in Caerphilly, South Wales and is married with two children.

Other books by Philip Burnard available from Chapman & Hall

Counselling Skills for Health Professionals
2nd edn (0 412 56690 7), 272 pages

Coping with Stress in the Health Professions
A handbook of experiential learning for health professionals
Paperback (0 412 38910 X), 208 pages

Personal Computing for Health Professionals
Paperback (0 412 49670 4), 256 pages

Health Care Computing
A survival guide for PC users
Paperback (0 412 60530 9), 224 pages

For more information, please contact:
The Promotion Department, Chapman & Hall,
2–6 Boundary Row, London SE1 8HN.

Writing for Health Professionals

A MANUAL FOR WRITERS

Second Edition

Philip Burnard

Reader, University of Wales College of Medicine, Cardiff, Wales.

CHAPMAN & HALL

London · Glasgow · Weinheim · New York · Tokyo · Melbourne · Madras

Published by Chapman & Hall, 2–6 Boundary Row, London SE1 8HN, UK

Chapman & Hall, 2–6 Boundary Row, London SE1 8HN, UK

Blackie Academic & Professional, Wester Cleddens Road, Bishopbriggs, Glasgow G64 2NZ, UK

Chapman & Hall GmbH, Pappelallee 3, 69469 Weinheim, Germany

Chapman & Hall USA, 115 Fifth Avenue, New York NY 10003, USA

Chapman & Hall Japan, ITP-Japan, Kyowa Building, 3F, 2-2-1 Hirakawacho, Chiyoda-ku, Tokyo 102, Japan

Chapman & Hall Australia, 102 Dodds Street, South Melbourne, Victoria 3205, Australia

Chapman & Hall India, R. Seshadri, 32 Second Main Road, CIT East, Madras 600 035, India

Distributed in the USA and Canada by Singular Publishing Group Inc., 4284 41st Street, San Diego, California 92105

First edition 1992
Reprinted 1994
Second edition 1996

© 1996 Philip Burnard

Typeset in 10/12pt Times by Saxon Graphics Ltd, Derby
Printed in Great Britain by St Edmundsbury Press Ltd, Bury St Edmunds, Suffolk

ISBN 0 412 71980 0   1 56593 172 6 (USA)

A catalogue record for this book is available from the British Library

Library of Congress Catalog Card Number: 95-71225

∞   Printed on permanent acid-free text paper, manufactured in accordance with ANSI/NISO Z39.48-1992 and ANSI/NISO Z39.48-1984 (Permanence of Paper).

For Sally, Aaron and Rebecca

Contents

Acknowledgements

Acknowledgements are offered to the British Standards Institution for permission to reproduce the proofreading marks and to Chapman & Hall for permission to reproduce the sample contract in the appendices of this book. Thanks, too, to the American Psychological Society for permission to reproduce the notes on non-sexist writing, also in the appendices. I am also grateful to Rob Heil of the Saint Maarten Medical Center Foundation, Saint Maarten, for supplying me with further material about referencing and to Martin Noble for editing this edition.

Trade names

The following registered trade names have been used in this book:

Animator, Applause, Apple, Apple Macintosh, Arts and Letters, Claris Works, Clean Sweep, Corel Draw, Dashboard, Dataease, dBase, Dream, EFMS, EndNote Plus, Excel, Excel for Windows, File Express, Findex 3×5, Flexbase, Freelance Graphics, Harvard Graphics, IBM Idealist, Idealist for Windows, Info Select, Infobase, Lotus, Mavis Beacon Teaches Typing, Memory Mate, Microsoft, Microsoft Access, Microsoft Office, Microsoft Project, Microsoft Publisher, Microsoft Works, Norton Utilities, Novell Office, Oxford Writer's Shelf, Page Plus, Page Wizards, Papers, Paradox, PC File, PC Tools, Q and A Write, R:Base, R:Base Personal, SmartSuite, Vault, Walkman, Windows, Word, Word for Windows, WordPerfect, WordPerfect for Windows, Zephyr.

Introduction

I try to leave out the parts that people skip.

Elmore Leonard

Like it or not, most health professionals have to write. In the last few years, this has become even more apparent. As health professionals of all sorts become more highly qualified, so they have to write more. Many carry out research projects and many more share their ideas through writing for publication. With the continuing development of the Internet – that sprawling but useful network of computer networks, many people are writing in a new, immediate way. The Internet allows health professionals to communicate around the world in seconds. It seems unlikely, though, that the Internet will replace the more formal written word: in papers, articles, books and records.

Non-fiction writing is more attractive when it is easy to read. It helps everyone if what you write is both easy and interesting to look at. Most of us can improve our writing. In this second edition of this book about writing, I have tried to expand the text to make it even more practical. For the sort of writing that health professionals most often do is of a **practical** nature. This book, then, is about non-fiction writing – writing so that other health professionals, teachers, patients and anyone else with whom we come in contact can make sense of what we think and do.

When you write a book like this you put yourself on the line. You run the risk of people reading what you have written and saying 'he is saying one thing and doing another'. You stand to break the rules that you set up – quite badly. That is probably not such a terrible thing. Besides, that should be part of the process of using this book. As you read it, notice when rules are broken. Check the phrasing, the sentence and paragraph construction and see whether or not I have stuck to the rules. Then see whether or not the rules would have improved the passage in question. Begin to read books as much for their style, layout and general format as for their content. If you are going to write, you need to see plenty of examples of all of these things: good, bad and indifferent.

In this second edition, I have generally revised and updated the text and added the following features:

- more practical examples of what is described in the text;
- more details about the writing process;
- information about punctuation and layout;
- descriptions of the Internet and of computer software useful to writers;
- sections on **reviewing** – books and other people's work;
- information about plagiarism and how to avoid it;
- information about copyright;
- examples of what other writers have said about writing.

A word about sexism and the writing process. I find the use of 'his or her' and its variants clumsy. I have decided to use 'her' to refer to the person who might be writing, throughout the book. Read 'his' where this applies to you. At present, there is no elegant way of avoiding sexism in writing but we should continue to work at it. There is an appendix to this book that illustrates ways in which sexism in writing **can** be avoided but some of the suggestions lead to some fairly ugly compromises.

WHO IS THIS BOOK FOR?

All health professionals have to write. Some enjoy doing it. Others loathe the thought of picking up a pen or sitting at a keyboard. This book is for a wide range of health professionals. I particularly hope it will be of use to the following groups of people:

- students in the health professions on certificate, diploma, undergraduate and postgraduate courses;
- researchers who have to write papers, dissertations or theses;
- practitioners in the clinical or community field who find themselves wanting or having to write;
- managers who have to prepare reports and are not sure how to;
- lecturers and teachers who want some ideas about advising students;
- the general reader who wants some straightforward ideas about how to write.

In a phrase: this book is for you. If you want to write, it will give you some practical help. It won't make writing easy, if you already find it difficult. But it might help.

WHAT IS IN THE BOOK?

In summary, this book aims to help you do the following things:
- write clearly and well;
- keep a bibliographic database;
- write essays;

- write articles;
- write books;
- write reviews;
- write research reports, dissertations and theses;
- write educational materials;
- choose a computer for writing;
- select the right software;
- use computers as an aid to writing;
- lay out and edit your work.

While almost anyone can write, there are certain rules that can make writing easier. Also, there are two keywords that I will often return to in this book. They are: **structure** and **simplicity**. If you want to writ; well, structure your work. If you want to be understood and want people to enjoy reading your work, keep it simple. Look at literature. Most modern literature is simply written. The most difficult things can be understood more easily if they are written clearly and simply. Wittgenstein, the philosopher, put this into one of his major philosophical works: 'What can be said at all can be said clearly: and whereof one cannot speak thereof one must be silent.'[1] Think about it. If it **can** be said at all, it can be said clearly. If it **cannot** be said, we are better off not trying to say it. That seems to me to sum up the issue.

Here, already, is an indication of the sort of observation I would like you to make. In the last paragraph, I used a footnote. Footnotes are not very popular these days and for good reason. Notice what the footnote made you do. You **had** to look down to the bottom of the page. In doing so, you probably lost your place and had to find it again. You probably forgot what I was busy writing about. First lesson: avoid footnotes like the plague. Also, avoid tired clichés. Unfortunately, you will note that I break both of these rules. That may be the second lesson: break the rules occasionally.

The first chapter deals with the basics: how to begin to write and how to structure your work. Then there is a chapter on the basic equipment you might need. The next two deal with the question of computing and using software. Chapter 5 tells you how to set up and use computer databases as an aid to writing. The following chapters consider specific sorts of writing: educational, essays, theses and dissertations, articles and books. You may find, once you start writing, that you progress through these different levels. You may, for example, start by having to write essays for a course. You might then write a very good one that someone advises you to send in for publication. Then, rather than taking the person at her word, you have work to do. You cannot just send in the essay as it stands. Chapter 9 will tell you how to modify it so that it may be published. There is a big difference between writing essays and writing articles.

1. Wittgenstein (1961).

If you get articles published, you may want to try writing a book. The health care field is a large one and there is always room for a new approach to an aspect of it. A book turns out to be like an article, only bigger. How much bigger? Read Chapter 10 and you will find out. Again, you will also find out how structure can help to make your ideas into a book. In Chapter 11, I explain how I write and hope that this summarizes what has gone before.

I hope that this book will help you in whatever sort of writing you have to do.

HOW DO I USE THE BOOK?

There are at least two ways to read this book. One is to start at the beginning and work your way through. This is obviously true of any book. So obviously true that many people think that this is the **proper** way to read a book. It is, if the book is a novel. With non-fiction, though, it is often more useful to browse through the contents page and the index and then to decide which parts of the book you are going to find most useful. Most non-fiction is best read in this way. It is rarely helpful to sit down (or worse – lie down) and read such a book from cover to cover. Instead, read selectively. I usually find that when I begin to read a book in this way I end up reading the whole book: but not in the order that the writer put the chapters together.

Also, if this is your book, make liberal use of a marker pen. Highlight the passages that are going to help you when you get down to your own writing. In the end, books are for using. That is why paperbacks are so much better than hardbacks. People are less reverent towards them. This can have at least two effects. First, readers are less likely to think that 'it must be right because it's in a book' – people become more critical.

Second, readers are less likely to feel that they must not write in the paragraphs or use marker pens. The reason that you can buy so many different sorts of marker pens is simply because there is a market for them. Buy a whole range and use them liberally. Only do this if you own the book. I hate bringing home library books and finding that a previous reader has added her own comments. Sometimes they are humorous in their extremity (awful book! don't read this page!) but in the end, they are annoying. Do write in your own books.

I have enjoyed writing and rewriting this book and I have learned a lot about writing in the process. I hope that you find it useful and wish you the best of luck with your own writing projects. Start writing now.

Philip Burnard
Caerphilly
Mid Glamorgan

'Oh,' said Helen Earle, polite but unimpressed. 'It must be wonderful to be a writer too. It's so very interesting.'

'It has its points,' he said ... he had thought for years it was a dog's life.

F. Scott Fitzgerald, *Afternoon of an Author*

Writing: the basics

My task is by the power of the written word to make you hear, to make you feel – it is, before all, to make you see.

Joseph Conrad

I notice that you use plain, simple language, short words and brief sentences. That is the way to write English. It is the modern way and the best way. Stick to it.

Mark Twain

An author called Ernest Gaines once wrote what he called the 'SixF Golden Rules of Writing': read, read, read and write, write, write. The simple rules are hard to better. The writer must read. Reading is the fuel for good writing whatever the writing might be for. If you are a health professional who is intending to write, it is likely that you already read. But what do you read? The literature in your field? Research reports? Business reports? Papers that you are referred to by your colleagues or teachers? The writer reads anything and everything. I think a good starting point for reading is to consider these areas:

- books related to your field;
- journal papers related to your area of interest;
- peripheral papers;
- magazines related to your field;
- newspapers;
- novels – especially literature;
- autobiographies;
- biographies;
- cereal packets and adverts.

In other words, try to read everything. It is all important fuel, however well or badly it may be written – and some of the worst writing comes in the academic journals. Be catholic and eclectic. Avoid limiting yourself to heavy books and papers in your field. Not only will you get bored but you will also find your own style quickly becomes stilted and dull. Buy the occasional magazine or journal from a field different to your own. When, for example, did you pick up or buy *The Grocer*? Have you ever read *Women's Weekly* or *Just Seventeen*? All magazines can teach you something about writing.

This does not mean, of course, that you have to be obsessional about the written word. Alan Bennett makes a nice, dry point about those who find themselves too attached to books:

> As for me, while I'm not baffled by books, I can't see how anyone can love them ('He loved books'). I can't see how anyone can 'love literature'. What does that mean? (Bennett, 1994)

You may not 'love' them, then, but it is important to read them.

This is the first rule: read as much as you can. Read for content. Read for structure and layout. Have a look through this book. Notice how it is laid out. How many blank lines are there between subheadings and text? Have you noticed details like that before? You will in future: if you intend to write. For the aim is to become a technically proficient writer as well as a 'good' writer. That means mastering some simple rules of layout and design and that is what this book will help you with. You may feel that this is obsessional attention to detail. I don't. I once sent in a manuscript to a heavyweight journal. I had made certain corrections to the typed manuscript and I had simply written them in with a pen. A few weeks later I received this dry comment in a letter of acceptance:

> Please pay more attention to the presentation of your manuscripts otherwise you may not be published in this journal again.

At first, I took offence and got very high-handed about the whole thing. What a nerve. Why should I have to be threatened in this way? After a while, though and after working as a journal reviewer myself, I came to appreciate what that rather direct editor had in mind. Presentation does matter. It is one thing to write ageless prose (and we are not likely to achieve that in a hurry). It is another to make sure that it is offered to the reader in a recognizable form. The more you write, the more important this becomes. Few book publishers will look favourably on a scrappily typed manuscript. It pays to think about what your finished work will look like on the page.

Notice how layout affects you. If you browse through a bookshop, you don't simply look at authors, titles or covers. You open the book and look through the pages. Why do you do that? Not only to pick up the gist of the book but also to see whether or not you like the layout. As you do this you will notice a number of things without really thinking about it. You will feel the quality of the paper.

You will notice how large or small the typeface is. You will notice whether or not words are crammed onto the page or laid out with plenty of 'white space'. It is an interesting and obscure fact that good layout in book printing calls for a ratio of 50% text to 50% of white space. This sounds unlikely but turns out to be true of most printed pages. If the page is more crammed with print than this, you are unlikely to find the book attractive.

In my view, the American publishers are better at dealing with the question of page layout than are UK publishers. Most American textbooks are studies in how to make the page and chapter look attractive. On the other hand, the British press is catching up fast. These sorts of concerns should become yours.

If you are writing essays for a course, you may feel that this does not apply to you. It does. As a university lecturer, I have to mark hundreds of essays every year. I always start with the best-looking ones. Not very academic you may say. Bear in mind that marking usually takes place late in the evening. It pays to humour the person who is marking your work and offer her something she will enjoy reading. It pays to write well and it pays to present your work well. Think carefully about the following issues:

- the paper that you write or print on;
- how you lay out your page;
- the typeface or 'font' that you use;
- the spacing between lines;
- how to make your work look uncluttered and clear;
- how many paragraphs you have on a page.

TYPES OF WRITING

There is a wide range of opportunities to write in the health professions. Opportunity is the right word here although some, as we have noted, see writing as a chore. Perhaps, like other skills, we enjoy writing more when we get better at it. Here are some examples of the opportunities to write:

- essays
- dissertations
- theses
- research reports
- abstracts
- journal articles
- journal papers
- books
- letters to the editor of journals
- short 'fillers' for magazines
- short articles for newsletters
- course materials

- curriculum packages
- advertising copy

The principles that are discussed throughout this book are applicable to all of these sorts of writings. If you hate writing, read on. You may get to like it. You may not, of course, but you may get better at it.

GETTING IDEAS

One thing is important here: you must have something to write about. I once borrowed an idea from the American poet Robert Lowell. I walked into a workshop on writing skills and gave the students instructions. All I said was: 'Write something.' Some got on with this straightaway. Others struggled to put two or three sentences together. The point is that you can write about anything. In the health professions there is always something to write about. If you cannot get inspired from the business of caring for other people, draw upon one or more of the following sources of inspiration:

- personal experience;
- working life;
- family and friends;
- unusual experiences;
- holidays;
- reading;
- TV;
- radio;
- visits abroad;
- sexual experiences;
- altered states of consciousness (through meditation etc.);
- other people's anecdotes;
- conferences;
- accidents;
- odd experiences;
- your imagination;
- the future;
- the past;
- the immediate present;
- how you wish things were;
- how you wish things were not;
- your beliefs;
- your values;
- your religious beliefs or lack of them.

It should be easy to add to this list. Writing consists mainly of having something to write about, then exercising some basic skills to get the ideas down on paper. I don't believe that there is anything magical about the process though I appreciate that some people write better and more easily than others.

QUALITY AND MEANING

Is some writing **better** than others? In my list of recommended reading, above, I have suggested that, alongside literature and journals, you read cereal packets. I have been asked by some readers if I mean this, for – surely – there are some forms of text that are better than others. From a post-modern point of view, however, there is **nothing** but the text (Docherty, 1993). Text is text is text. It is all black marks on white pages. We, as readers, 'invent' the meaning of the text and – if you like – the 'reader writes the text'. This particularly liberal point of view acknowledges that what is common to all forms of writing is words and words arranged on the page. In this sense, then, **all** writing is an attempt to communicate and there is never only **one** meaning attached to what is written. As we read Shakespeare, we bring our own meanings to bear. As we read slogans in advertisements, we also 'read in' our own interpretations of what the advertisers meant. All of this makes it difficult to begin to talk about an absolute yardstick for quality in writing.

On the other hand, if we are to discuss 'rules of writing' – and this book is about those – then it is being acknowledged that certain rules **are** possible. As always, it is useful to take in a **range** of points of view – about writing as about other things – and the post-modern view can be useful in thinking differently about writing, quality and meaning.

RULES OF GOOD WRITING

Robert Gunning (1968) offers ten principles of clear writing:

- keep sentences short;
- prefer the simple to the complex;
- prefer the familiar word;
- avoid unnecessary words;
- put action in your verbs;
- write like you talk;
- use terms your reader can picture;
- tie in with your reader's experience;
- make full use of variety;
- write to express not impress.

It is worth considering each of these in turn and the reader is also referred to Gunning's book. It is a readable and important analysis of how to write well.

Keep sentences short

This speaks for itself. Short sentences (and short paragraphs) are easy on the eye and easy to read. Many people loose the thread of long sentences. Try to get into the habit of halving all of your sentences that are more than about six or seven words in length. Most people's writing can benefit from editing in this way. Also avoid too many lists that end in 'and'. Instead, deal with each item separately. On the other hand, don't try to make all your sentences the same length. Too many short sentences can be a distraction. Use two or three short ones and then use a slightly longer one. Vary your sentence and paragraph length a little. If in doubt, though, keep them short. Consider these three examples and see if what I have written makes sense to you:

Example 1.1a
Most people have to write. Many write for courses. I have completed a number of courses. All required essays. Some wanted long essays. Others wanted short. I found the early ones difficult. Writing got easier later on. Now I enjoy writing. Not everyone does. I wonder if you do.

Example 1.1b
It is probably true that most people have to write at some time in their life. Many people have to write essays for courses and they have all sorts of things to consider when they do this: they have to think about planning their work; they have to find somewhere to write and they have to consider how to integrate their work with their social life. While social life is important to most people it should not interfere with your studies and if you can, you should avoid mixing the pub with your essay writing activities.

Example 1.1c
Most people have to write. Students usually have to write essays for courses. Essay writing, while not difficult, takes some planning. The key issue is outlining. A simple outline can save time. Most people, once they have learned to outline, find that they can write much more easily. Experimentation may be the answer. Try writing with outlines. Try writing without. If you find that the outlining process helps, keep at it. If not, stop.

Example 1.1a shows the use of short sentences. While it is readable, the style is rather staccato. Example 1.1b illustrates how long sentences can be awkward and difficult to follow. Example 1.1c shows the use of both short and longer sentences. Hopefully, the third example is the easiest to read. Also, the sudden use of a very short sentence can be used to heighten dramatic effect. Note, for example, the terse use of the final sentence in Example 1.1c.

Look through some of your own work and edit it. Cut out the lists of items separated by commas and shorten some of the sentences. Then read through your work and see whether or not you agree that shorter sentences make for clearer reading.

Prefer the simple to the complex

Do not try to be clever. Your readers will not appreciate it. Stick to ordinary words and do not try to confuse. As one lecturer at university told me: 'Anyone who has anything interesting to say will not risk being misunderstood.' Some students on courses are tempted to use flowery language in the belief that it will sound 'academic'. Some academics are tempted this way too. This is fine if you are writing an academic monograph to be read by a handful of other people. Most of us are not (and even in a monograph, simple and clear language is to be preferred).

Consider the following two examples of text written about the same subject but in rather different ways.

Example 1.2a
There is a sense in which all of us can appreciate the universality of the human condition. Whilst, in a sense, we are all unique, so too do we share – in very real ways – a variety of features of considerable similitude. In our being grounded in the very substance of humanity we are able to project outwards and reach out to those with whom we share that humanity.

Example 1.2b
We are similar to each other in some ways. In other ways, we are unique. What is personal is also universal.

I suggest that the second example says much the same as the first but is much simpler and easier to understand. The first example is also full of 'academic' redundancies such as 'there is a sense in which' – a phrase that really means very little.

Strong (1991) says this about simple writing:

> Writing simply and clearly is not easy. Anne Tyler writes that 'it's hard to be simple, the hardest thing there is'. On the other hand, direct writing *feels* right. 'When I see a paragraph shrinking under my eyes like a strip of bacon in a skillet', Peter De Vries says, 'I know I'm on the right track'. (Strong, 1991)

Prefer the familiar word

Use words that everyone knows. Don't use 'notion' when you mean 'idea'. Avoid 'pedestrian' when you mean boring. And so on. Most of us have words that we **enjoy** using. Be careful of them. A famous writer in the last century wrote that whenever he came upon a passage in his work that he particularly liked, he crossed it out. We can easily fool ourselves that we are writing ever-lasting prose. Mostly, we are not. Keep it simple. Or, as the Americans would have it: observe the KISS principle. Keep it simple, stupid. In a similar but different vein, Gillett offers the following advice on finding the 'right' words:

> The right words are those that are: concrete rather than abstract, short rather than long, familiar rather than unfamiliar, direct rather than round-about, economical rather than flowery. (Gillett, 1990)

On the other hand, none of this means that you have to be **boring**. It is important to continue to explore words and their meanings. Sixty years ago, Dorothea Brande had this to say:

> Be on the alert to find appropriate words wherever you read, but before you use them be sure they are congruous when side by side with words of your own vocabulary. Combing a thesaurus for what an old professor of mine used to call, contemptuously, 'vivid verbs' will be far less useful than to find words in the midst of a living story; although a thesaurus is a good tool if it is used as it is meant to be. (Brande, 1934)

Avoid unnecessary words

Another straightforward one. Try to cut out the 'howevers' and the 'neverthe-lesses'. Avoid qualifying adjectives with 'very' (as in: it is very important that student social workers ...). Especially avoid **double** qualification ('very, very').

I have a soft spot for the word 'vital'. If I am not careful, I find myself writing tired old sentences that start: 'It is vital that health professionals ...'. As you read through this book, notice how often I use the word. Hopefully, you won't find it at all. Having acknowledged my overuse of it, I have tried to prune it out. Try to do this with your own favourites. Note, too, that with a word processor, it is easy to seek out these 'favourites' and put in other, more varied, words. The **search and replace** feature helps you to do this.

Put action in your verbs

Action gets people moving. Words like 'go' and 'move' keep people reading. Try to make your writing active rather than passive. There is still a tendency in the academic world for everything to be written in the past tense. Try breaking that rule. Also, avoid clumsy locutions (!) such as these: 'The writer feels that

...' or 'The current author acknowledges that ...' It is better to write 'I think that ...' After all, it must be clear that **you** are the writer or author. If not, who?

Write like you talk

This is an important one but one that is easily ignored. The statement itself is an example of 'writing like you talk'. More grammatically, it should be 'write as you talk'. But who would **say** something like: 'I feel that it is of considerable importance that clients in the health profession are offered the provision of counselling'? No one. If you tend to write in this way, try clipping those sorts of sentences down like this: 'People should be offered counselling when they want it.' Much clearer. The test of whether or not you are observing this rule is to read out what you have written. If you would not say it, do not write it. This applies to both fiction and non-fiction.

This is, I appreciate, a contentious issue. Not everyone will want to write like they speak and nor will everyone want **others** to write like **they** speak. A lot will depend on the sort of language style that the writer adopts in everyday life. Clearly, the following would not be a very acceptable style of writing in an academic essay:

> It's, like, Freud described the unconscious. He can't have been the first. After all, there must have been an unconscious before Freud arrived – but you get what I mean: he was the first, as far as we know, to put it all into words. He seemed to have known what he was on about, if you get my drift.

Clairborne (1990), in a study of the use of the English language, cites some examples of some **particularly** badly written material, from American sources:

- A first-year college student: 'It's obvious, in our modern world of today, there's a lot of impreciseness in expressing thoughts we have.'
- A candidate for an M.A. at a large Midwestern university: 'If you know the problems, the children are difficult to evaluate with.'
- A doctor: 'Symptomatology relative to impending or incipient onset of illness generally manifests itself initially via a marked chill, followed by a rapid rise of temperature to the 103 degree – 105 degree range is characteristically observed.'
- A teacher (!) writing to a parent: 'Scott is dropping in his studies he acts as if he don't Care. Scott want pass in his assignment at all, he had a poem to learn and he fell tu do it.'
- A book review in the *New Yorker*: 'If he were trying to pull himself together by hanging on to Esther's sanity, and she knew that and parlayed it, there would be come dynamics and edges.' (Clairborne, 1990)

What Gunning was suggesting, though, was that there is no need to use **complicated** language in writing. When we write, we often use a lot of padding that we do not use in speech. The 'read it out loud' principle, described above, is a good way of weeding out the superfluities.

Use terms your reader can picture

Try to use metaphors and illustrations that create pictures for the reader. Just because you are writing a report does not mean that you cannot 'illustrate' your writing in this way. Be careful, though. Make sure that you do not mix metaphors. This, apart from being grammatically wrong (which is not a big problem) causes all sorts of problems with imagery. My favourite mixed metaphor is one I heard a psychiatrist use: 'We all leaned over backwards to oil the wheels for this patient.' Oddly enough, this is a mixed metaphor that you **can** picture but the picture is a strange one.

On this sort of issue, avoid 'the screamer'. The screamer is the writing trade's name for the exclamation mark. If something is funny or ironic, the reader will notice. You don't have to rub their nose in it. If you do use an exclamation mark, only ever use one. Never use two or three!!! Keep multiple exclamation marks for reminder notes you leave yourself on the top of the TV to remember to pay the milkman.

Tie in with your reader's experience

Illustrate what you write with small 'case studies' or illustrations from life. Invite the reader to think of her own examples of what you are talking about. At the same time, avoid rhetorical questions. It is irritating to read questions that seem to hang in the air without an answer. Isn't it?

Make full use of variety

If you can, use things to help your reader to keep awake. If you are writing an article for a journal, use checklists and boxed 'word illustrations'. This helps to break up large chunks of text. Look through any magazine that you have to hand. What you will find is that only the academic journals use continuous blocks of text. All others use variety to keep the reader interested. On the other hand, don't use these devices for their own sake. Make sure that they add to the reader's understanding of your writing.

Write to express not impress

This is the ultimate point. Your aim is not to show how clever you are. It should be to communicate your ideas to other people. This point seems to summarize all of the other ones. Many students, when they start to write essays for diploma and degree courses, think that they have to try to imitate the worst sorts of academic writing. Perhaps they read journal papers in fairly dull journals. Perhaps some of their lecturers talk in that way. Whatever the reason, the point is to stop writing in that fashion. Write simply, clearly and use the obvious word rather than the more complicated. Consider the following extract from a nursing book and think about whether or not it could have been written more clearly (you may even want to consider what it **means**):

> The ability to engage in self-care is also conceptualized as having form and content. Self-care agency is conceptualized as taking the form of a set of human abilities for deliberate action: the ability to attend to specific things (this includes the ability to exclude other things) and to understand their characteristics and the meaning of the characteristics; the ability to apprehend the need to change or regulate the things observed; the ability to acquire knowledge of appropriate courses of action for regulation; the ability to decide what to; and the ability to act to achieve change or regulation. The content of self-care agency derives from its proper object, meeting self-care requisites, whatever those requisites are at specific moments. (Orem, 1980)

George Orwell, in his 1946 book *Politics and the English Language*, quoted in the *Economist Pocket Style Book* (1986), offered a similar but different list of recommendations. While Orwell's 'six elementary rules' offer similar advice to Gunning's, they also highlight some other important, stylistic issues:

1. Never use a metaphor, simile or other figure of speech which you are used to seeing in print.
2 Never use a long word where a short word will do.
3. If it is possible to cut out a word, always cut it out.
4. Never use the passive where you can use the active.
5. Never use a foreign phrase, a scientific word or a jargon word if you can think of an everyday English equivalent.
6. Break any of these rules sooner than say anything outright barbarous.

Writing, then, should be fresh, straightforward and well constructed. There is no need to use difficult words, foreign phrases for effect or unnecessary jargon. In the next section, we explore jargon.

THE USE OF JARGON

Interestingly – and no doubt, correctly – almost any book you read about writing stresses the need for **simplicity**. The suggestion is usually that sentences and paragraphs should be short and that the simpler word should be preferred to the more complicated. And yet it is possible to pick up very many medical texts and find complicated, not to say impenetrable writing. Hudson (1978) in his book *The Jargon of the Professions* identifies the sorts of writers that are particularly at risk from using complicated and jargon-ridden writing. According to Hudson, they are:

- Those who are insecure and who feel they must do everything possible to make society feel that it needs their services.
- Those who are ashamed of what they do and are driven to find suitable language with which to gild their activities.
- Those who need big words, as they need big cars, to give them an extra ration of size.
- Those who have nothing really to sell, and who need jargon in order to hoodwink the customers

In these consumer-driven days, it is to be hoped that, in the health care professions, no one is trying to 'hoodwink the customers'. Some health care writers may, however, be tempted to hoodwink each other with complicated language and with wild abstractions.

On the other hand, there is also an 'up' side to jargon. In certain research papers and articles submitted to learned journals, a small amount of jargon may be used as a shorthand. If it is known that a piece of writing is going to be read by an audience of limited size and made up of like-minded professionals then it may be useful to use a certain amount of jargon. Clearly, it would be impractical to explain and define **every** term in these circumstances. The objection to jargon is when it is being used for the reasons discussed in the previous paragraphs.

ABSTRACTION

Abstractions are popular. They are hard to refute and often lead to the writer sounding more clever than he or she really is – it also allows them to live in the clouds. Sir Ernest Gowers, in a classic book about clear writing had this to say about the use of abstract words:

> Unfortunately the very vagueness of abstract words is one of the reasons for their popularity. To express one's thoughts accurately is hard work, and to be precise is sometimes dangerous. We are tempted to prefer the safer obscurity of the abstract. It is the greatest vice of present-day writing. (Gowers, 1962)

And that was more than thirty years ago.

This is not to suggest that abstracts should **never** be discussed but, perhaps, to note that even abstract ideas should be grounded in reality. In practical professions such as the medical and paramedical professions, it would seem vital that **ideas** about those professions link very much with 'real life'. Sadly, a reading of some of the health care journals does not always bear out this direct relationship.

Complicated writing is sometimes encouraged by some academics' persistence in recommending the 'third person' as the only appropriate tense in academic writing. It has become a cliché in education that, for some reason, students completing courses should always avoid 'I' or 'we' in their writing. Instead, they should offer peculiar locutions such as 'in the present writer's view' or 'in the opinion of this author'. Who, if not 'I', is writing these words?

THIRD PERSON

The injunction to use the 'third person' is based on the fallacy that 'this is how academics write'. Kirkman (1992) in a survey of 81 academic journals from a wide range of disciplines – and all peer reviewed – found that only **seven** did not contain papers in which 'I', 'we' or 'our' featured. Put the other way, 74 academic journals **allowed** the use of these. Included in the list that **did** allow this usage was perhaps the most prestigious journal of all – *Nature*. None of this means that papers and articles have to be a litany of 'I's but just to acknowledge that if it is simpler to say 'I' then it is probably better.

Following Gunning (1968), there is a very simple test to see whether or not your writing is clear and simple. You read it out loud. If you find yourself thinking 'I would never **say** that', then the writing can probably be rephrased. After all, in speech – as we have noted – we would not be **allowed** to get away with being too complicated. In speech, we are likely to be challenged. Our writing, then, should imitate our speech. We should seek the transparent, the clear and the uncomplicated. Grammar – as Gowers was at pains to point out – should be a **guide** to writing, not an immutable law.

This is not to say that nothing written should ever be **complex**. It is quite possible to convey complex ideas clearly. Unfortunately, too often, it is the person who has little that is complex to say who wraps his or her ideas up in language (Kirkman, 1992). This, then, is not a call for reducing everything to its lowest common denominator – far from it. It is a call for clear writing.

In the end, of course, words and meanings are slippery. Just as we think we have written something that is unambiguous, someone else will come along and ask us what we mean. The production of a completely clear piece of writing is probably something out of reach. On the other hand, an examination of how we communicate **orally** gives us a clue to how we understand other people. Orally, we tend to work in approximations. We **think** we understand the other person and work on the basis that we have until the other person indicates otherwise. With writing, of course, there is no 'second chance' – the author is no longer around to explain any mistakes nor to clarify meanings. However, most of us don't read **every word** in a book, nor do we work through passages a word at a time. Instead, we build up an **impression** of what the writer means. Indeed, some fiction depends on this process. This is probably the best we can hope for – even in non-fiction. We should not, though, make the job any more difficult than it is already. Our aim, I maintain, is to write as clearly as we can and that almost always means **simply**. We all work with two vocabularies: an active one (the one we use in everyday life) and a passive one (which contains words we understand but don't use very often).

Note that the passive vocabulary often contains more than its fair share of abstract terms and may contain many 'approximations'. By 'approximations' I mean those words about which we have an idea of their meaning but would be hard pushed to pin down. What, for example, do the words 'phenomenology', 'positivism', 'paradigm' and 'humanism' **really** mean? My guess is that lots of different people would give you lots of different definitions – and many would claim to be right! Accessing the active vocabulary is likely to make both you and the reader more inclined to read on than if you are always tugging at your own and the readers' passive vocabulary.

The psychologist, David Canter, makes an interesting observation about the changing nature of words and – in particular – about the turning of nouns into verbs. Writing about the jargon attached to the psychology of crime, he writes:

> The term 'offender profiling' has stuck; yet another example of the admirably creative but infuriatingly confusing American reinvention of English words and phrases. Often the key to these word inventions is to take a noun in common use, preferably a noun that is reasonably abstract and is therefore used to describe a relatively complex phenomenon, such as 'police', 'priority' or 'interface', and to turn these into verbs where none existed before. A rather unclear notion emerges, rich in resonance: 'to police', 'to prioritize', 'to interface'. Now with skilled prestidigitation the verb can creep back in as a noun, but now it is describing a process: 'policing', 'prioritizing', 'interfacing'. Because of its roots in a reasonably specific well-known noun the impression is created that a distinct process exists that can be cut and dried and sold by the pound. (Canter, 1994)

On the other hand, you may want to take Canter to task for using words like 'prestidigitation'.

AVOID 'SIC'

The word '*sic*' is sometimes put in brackets after a direct quotation from someone else's work. It is there to indicate that the current writer acknowledges that the passage is not quite right, grammatically or in terms of spelling or structure. What it can **convey** is something like this:

> I realize, of course, that this is not how you or I would write but I am clever enough to bring to your notice that I have spotted the writer's error. Like you, I would not make the same mistake in my own writing. In future, be cautious about everything this writer has to say. He might

make similar mistakes again. He is not very reliable: keep his work at arm's length.

In other words, the use of '*sic*' can sound smug. It is best avoided if at all possible. There are times when you need to indicate that an unusual form of words was used. If you are writing up a research report that calls for direct quotations from interviews, then you need to use the respondent's own words. All you have to do, here, is to acknowledge, at an early stage in your report that you are offering direct quotations. You don't have to pepper your report with '*sic*'. An appropriate word if ever there was one.

KEEPING A JOURNAL

Consider keeping a writing journal. Many people start writing a diary, fill it in for a few days or weeks and then abandon it. Call yours a journal and keep on filling it in. Buy a large spiral or hardbound notebook. Put a label on the front and then use the following headings to organize your entries:

- New ideas for writing
- Longer term goals for research or books
- Quotations (including full reference and page number)
- New references
- Notes about self (Keep a note of your productivity versus your mood. Some people write better when they are slightly miserable. Writing can be cathartic.)
- Writing completed. (It is useful for your CV to have a running tally of the completed pieces of written work. This is particularly true if you have articles published in journals or magazines.)

Carry the journal with you at all times, if you can. Keep it by your bed and don't be afraid of jotting down ideas in the middle of the night. It you don't jot them down then, the ideas will often be gone by the morning.

Every so often, perhaps once a month, read through your journal. Pull out the references and put them in your bibliographical database. See whether or not you want to pursue the ideas for articles and file away your new quotations. Sometimes, the quotations can be put in the references database.

Keep this sort of journal for at least six months. After that, it tends to become something of a habit. It is certainly a more reliable way of keeping track of your thoughts and ideas than jotting them down on the backs of envelopes. Even if writing on the backs of envelopes seems rather more romantic.

Take some time in choosing the sort of book that you will use for your journal. This sort of hunting down is not only pleasurable in itself but it helps to reinforce the idea that you are serious about keeping the journal. Write for yourself but ponder about this thought from a friend of mine in the book trade.

He feels that **all** writing is biographical and a form of exhibitionism. Consider your own views on this and reread something that you have read. To what degree does that writing contain a part of you?

Also, consider **why** you write. I have suggested that writing may be cathartic. That is to say that it may be one way of our dealing with hidden conflicts and emotional stress. I don't want to be too psychological about all this. It is easy to dream up theories about why people do or don't do various things. Often, such theories are fairly spurious. It does seem to be true, however, that some forms of writing can be compulsive. Malcolm Bradbury has warned of how easy it can be to 'write yourself to death'. Hopefully, not too many of us do this. It is interesting, though, to ponder on one's motives for writing. Not for long, though. Much more important is the production of readable and hopefully saleable copy.

WRITING HABITS

I find it useful to be slightly ritualistic about writing. I try to write every day and I tend to start writing at much the same time. Brande, writing of the need to write regularly and to order suggests the following:

> After you have dressed, sit down for a moment by yourself and go over the day before you. Usually you can tell accurately enough what its demands and opportunities will be; roughly, at the least, you can sketch out for yourself enough of your program to know when you will have a few moments to yourself. It need not be very long; fifteen minutes will do nicely ... Decide for yourself when you will take that time for writing; for you are going to write in it ... Now this is very important, and can hardly be emphasized too strongly: *you have decided to write at four o'clock, and at four o'clock write you must! No excuses can be given.* (Brande, 1934)

First, I read through what I finished the evening before and then I carry on. I don't edit anything until I have finished the whole of a project and I try not to keep crossing out. I feel that it is important to develop a sense of flow. Although it has been said that what is easy to produce is unlikely to make easy reading, I feel that the opposite can also be true. If you slave for hours over every word you can end up with pages of stilted and difficult to read text. This is the odd paradox: you have to be careful about what you write but not so careful that it interferes with what you want to say.

If you want to check how readable your work is, consider investing in one of the Shareware programs that will 'read' and comment on your work. Usually, such programs offer you a 'FOG rating' index – a measure of how readable your work is (most of the larger word-processing programs also have a feature that will do this for you, too). As a rule, it is short sentences and simple words that win the day in the readability stakes. When you string together lengthy prose, you lose your reader. If necessary, go back and break up sentences with full stops. I often find this to be necessary. I have a habit of dividing sentences with colons. I can nearly always go back and replace the colon with a full stop. Colons, semi-colons and other such 'complicated' punctuation should be used sparingly.

STYLE

This is the most difficult thing of all to define. Style is not content. It refers to the way in which words are put together. Kirkman (1992) defines it like this:

> Style in writing is concerned with choice. Every writer has available the enormous resources of a whole language. English presents a particularly large range of choices of individual words, and of combinations of words into small and large 'structures' – idioms, phrases, clauses, sentences, paragraphs, sections, chapters. The choices we make create the 'style', which is a term covering balance, emphasis and tone. (Kirkman, 1992)

Like other sorts of reading, it is worth learning to read for style. This is easier with fiction than with non-fiction. Style is, however, present in non-fiction even if it is almost buried by the content. Too often, the style in non-fiction slips by us because we are caught up with the content. On the other hand, we **do** notice the style in that we readily dismiss that book as 'bad' and this one as 'easy to read'. The hardest thing of all is to begin to notice your own style. There is something paradoxical here. If you work at developing a style, you are likely to lose it. You begin to turn out pieces that are self-conscious. Try, instead, to forget your own style but work away at getting the following things in order:

- sentence construction;
- paragraph construction;
- use of new metaphors;
- clear use of description;
- interesting reporting of research;
- ability to inspire the reader;
- enough 'padding' between hard facts to keep the reader reading.

This last point may not be completely obvious. We cannot keep throwing fact after fact at the reader. In between chunks of facts, we need to have a little relief. This can come as criticism or commentary on what has gone before. Notice how other writers use this. Do not be tempted to pare down your style of writing so much that you leave out any sort of padding. On the other hand, be wary of page-filling for the sake of it. Lecturers and tutors who have to mark essays will be very aware of student's attempts at such page-filling. Take, for example, the following:

All health professionals, almost by definition, have to care. The whole process of caring is important in that it shows how a relationship between one person and another can develop in very meaningful ways. If we do not care we cannot be seen as real professionals nor can we be seen as true carers. Most health care workers prefer to see their work as having professional elements to it. Perhaps the caring aspect is the most important element of all. The question remains, however, how do we define care and what research has been done on the topic? These questions and many others are the subject of this essay. Essentially, it is vital that we fully appreciate the metaparadign that lies behind the philosophy of care that the health professional is offering vis à vis the client.

In offering advice to sub-editors, Jill Baker (1987) discusses the following basic rules of style:

- rewrite long sentences;
- replace pompous or polysyllabic words with simpler ones;
- make sure that the author's sentence construction is clear;
- omit unnecessary adjectives and omit qualifications such as 'very';
- ensure that words are used precisely;
- make sure that verbs are active;
- make sure that the author uses metaphors correctly and sparingly;
- replace jargon with a phrase in everyday use.

Finally, you must **care** about what you write. Writing is rarely a simple, mechanical process. When it is, it is usually **obvious** to the reader. Strong (1991) sums this up as follows:

Caring about what you write is the starting point. If *you* don't care about what you say and how you say it, why should anyone else? An indifferent attitude almost guarantees that no one will take you seriously. Communication in writing is like any human relationship: Nothing important or interesting happens unless you really care. (Strong, 1991)

PUNCTUATION

Like it or not, you need to get punctuation right. This is especially true if you are submitting work for examination or assessment. If you are sending in a manuscript for publication, the chances are that a sub-editor will help to modify your punctuation if it is wrong. On the other hand, you are less likely to have your work accepted for publication if your punctuation is obviously poorly used. It is worth considering Carey's comments on the use of punctuation:

Stops should be used as sparingly as sense will permit: but in so far as they are needed for an immediate grasp of the sense or for the avoidance of any possible ambiguity, or occasionally to relieve a very lengthy passage, they should be used as freely as need be. The best punctuation is that of which the reader is least conscious; for when punctuation, or the lack of it, obtrudes itself, it is usually because it offends. (Carey, 1976)

Here are some general pointers about punctuating.

- **Full stop** (.) Used at ends of sentences. Called a 'period' in North America. As in: 'I'm broke. Period.'
- **Comma** (,) Used between phrases, within sentences and in lists. As in 'He was tall, dark and extremely ugly.' Or: 'We sent them dates, prunes and pineapples.'
- **Semi-colon** (;) Used, in long sentences, to break up sections. It is often better to insert a full stop rather than use a semi colon. Examples: She walked on her hands as part of the circus performance; sometimes she stood in for one of the clowns. Or: She walked on her hands as part of the circus performance. Sometimes she stood in for one of the clowns.
- **Colon** (:) Used at the end of one phrase and the beginning of another, for emphasis or as the introduction to a list. Examples: 'The room was almost full: it would have been difficult to pack in any more people.' 'When you go on holiday, you may want to consider taking the following: your passport, money, something to read.'
- **Dash** (–) Used to insert a phrase into a sentence, almost as an 'aside', e.g. 'Fresh fish is a good buy – as are sausages – for the person who wants a cheap meal.'
- **Inverted commas** (" ") Used around speech and, sparingly, to highlight a word or phrase, sometimes with irony. Not to be overused as a means of emphasis, e.g. 'Don't call me that!' she said, obviously angry. He was 'gutted' by the response he got following the distribution of the questionnaires.
- **Exclamation mark** (!) Used – and overused – as a form of exclamation or emphasis. Sometimes used to indicate that a sentence is meant to be funny. If it is, it should stand up for itself, without the exclamation mark. If in doubt, do not use an exclamation mark.

If in doubt, keep punctuation simple. Use full stops rather than colons and semi-colons to break up text. Instead of using lots of commas, put in a full stop, instead. Begin to notice how other people use punctuation. Start, if you like, by looking at the way it is used in this book.

PRACTICE WRITING

There are certain exercises that you can do to improve your writing. First, try the process know as 'free writing'. Get up every morning and sit down at the computer keyboard. Then begin to type. Type anything that comes into your head. At first, do not attempt to disallow anything that comes to mind. The aim is to get as much writing done in the shortest time possible. Start by doing this for two minutes and build up to doing it for ten minutes. As you get better at it, begin to pay attention to the form and content of the writing. Do not go to the keyboard with a specific idea in mind but gradually, as ideas come to you, begin to quickly work them into shape. Do all this without prior planning and without doing an outline for what you are writing. Here is an example of free writing:

```
It's cold in here and I have to write about groups.
The important thing about groups is facilitation.
Probably. Possibly. Perhaps the most important thing
about groups is being in one. Think of groups that I
have been in. Where do I start? Groups from school-
days: classes, cubs, scouts and so on. Groups from
teenage years: friends, parties. Professional groups.
Not that I belong to any at the moment. Should I join
one? Why do people join groups? Sometimes, of course,
they have no choice. Primary and secondary groups:
note the differences. Is there anyone out there who
does not belong to some group or other? I doubt it.
Even the ones that weren't in groups would be members
of a group called 'people who don't live in groups'.
What a thought: no escape.
```

This exercise is one of the best ones for dealing with writer's block and it is also excellent for encouraging you to work quickly. Later on (or even sooner) you may be asked to write a column for a magazine in your profession. If you do that, you will have to write quickly. Often, you will be asked for about 1000 words by the end of the week. You have no choice, then. You have to write quickly. Keep this exercise going for a few weeks or consider keeping it going all the time. John Braine, the author, found this activity a particularly useful one for helping him to work quickly and accurately.

The other activity consists of editing a passage of writing (Figure 1.1). Read through the passage and consider how you could improve it. Pay attention, particularly to the following points:

- sentence and paragraph construction;
- phrasing;
- use of words;
- any unnecessary words or phrases;
- the flow of the piece.

As you work through this activity, consider the style of the piece. Did you enjoy reading it? Was it lively? Did it have zest? Did you want to read more?

The term 'health professional' covers a multitude of sins: health professionals can range from occupational therapists, to doctors and from nurses to other sorts of health care workers, although not everyone likes that label. What distinguishes health care professionals from other sorts of health care workers? This is an important question and one that demands to be answered soon if we are to offer a viable and healthy service to patients, clients, residents and other consumers of care. Perhaps it is the word 'professional'. The word 'professional' has many connotations and many meanings. It means different things to different people. To some it means one thing and to others it means something else. In this paper, I plan to consider the word 'professional' and try to identify what it means as it relates to the health professions. The term 'professional' is widely used to describe widely differing sorts of occupations and jobs. For example, it is possible to talk about 'professional footballers' but no one would, normally, compare professional footballers to, say, lawyers who are also professionals but different sorts of professionals. Some writers have attempted to identify the sorts of criteria that can be used to distinguish professionals from non-professionals and these methods will be discussed in the next few paragraphs. What is important from the point of view of the health care professional is also to look at the literature on health care and trace the history of those workers to the present day in which the idea of professionalization has become an important issue.

Figure 1.1 Text to edit.

If not, consider why not. Make the changes that you would make if you were being asked to publish the piece in a newspaper or magazine. Your task is to make the passage readable and interesting. As you do this, notice to what degree your own writing problems are contained in the passage. Do you fall into the traps that this writer did or are your shortcomings different ones? Part of the process of becoming an effective writer is to know something about your own style of writing. It is often possible to see it reflected in the writings of others. That is why it is useful to be asked to be a reviewer for a journal or magazine. You are unlikely to be paid for the task but it will quickly teach you what editors do and do not accept as suitable copy for publication.

On that point, read a variety of health care journals and compare their styles. Some will make full use of subheadings (often of the single-word variety). These tend to be used to break up solid blocks of text. The more academic journals presumably assume that their readers have more staying power. They use fewer headings and the headings tend to be more descriptive and accurate. Few journals or magazines have no subheadings at all. Notice, too, how paragraphs are laid out in magazines and journals. Because most are printed in double columns, editors tend to prefer short paragraphs. In double column layout, these are easier to read. Try to spot exceptions to this rule. Sometimes, an editor of an academic journal will not do substantial editing to a particular paper. Often, such papers will have longer paragraphs than usual. As ever, the nearer you can get your own work to the publishable standard, the better it is likely to be. It is quite easy to learn the basics of layout.

SIMPLICITY AND STRUCTURE

These remain the keywords. All the best writing is simple in style. All the best writing is structured. A simple writing style is not always easy to achieve. It can be made easier, though, if you try to avoid 'fillers' such as the following:

- there is a sense in which ...
- however ...
- it is the writer's view that ...
- it is sometimes the case that ...
- the writer would like to forward the view that ...
- We have to consider this over and against the other view that ...

All of these hide the message. Sometimes academics use them to try to hedge their bets. It is as if they are saying to the reader: 'I know there are other points of views and this may not be the right one and that there are a whole range of other things that could be said here but ...' In the end, we have to be prepared to stick to what we want to say and say it. It really is as simple as that. Mostly we are not writing philosophy so we don't have to ponder over every nuance of meaning and possibility. Take some risks. Declare what you want to say without the wrapping. But ... keep it structured.

COUNTING WORDS

A professional writer counts words. She has to. Most professionals are paid according to the number of words they write. Most professionals, too, are told the limit of the words they can write. This book, for example, should be about 75–85 000 words in length. If I wrote 120 000 words, the editor would probably complain and might send the manuscript back. If I wrote 200 000 words, she certainly would. If, on the other hand, I sent in a manuscript of 35 000 words, she would send that back too. There is little margin for negotiation once limits have been set. This is also true for essays, dissertations and projects. Find out the limit and then work to it but don't go over it. Also, the discipline of working to a set number of words can tighten up your style. **Prefer** to work to a word limit and see the development of your writing. You can say a lot in 1000 words and a lot in 100 000.

THE REAL BASICS

Michael Larson (1986) offers the following checklist for prospective writers. His list (which includes an essential American book about writing) is appropriate to all would-be writers in the health professions. He maintains that all writers should have:

- Something to say
- The compulsive need to say it
- Talent: the gift for turning ideas into words, characters, and the situations, and knowing when they are right
- Discipline
- Persistence
- Faith in your work
- Trust in your instincts
- Patience with your talents and others' appreciation of it
- Reading
- *The Elements of Style*, by William Strunk, Jr. and E. B. White
- The need to grow as a writer and the experience with art and life to do so. (Larson, 1986)

The next book to read is Strunk and White.

Equipment and environment

The bookful blockhead, ignorantly read,
With loads of learned lumber in his head.

Alexander Pope

Most of the people I know seem to like buying stationery. There is something attractive about the pads and files in W. H. Smith's. This chapter identifies some of the equipment you may want to consider if you are going to write. It will be a short chapter. These days, the basic and most important item of equipment is the computer. If you want to write and you do not have one: buy one. It will change the way you write, conclusively.

WHERE TO WRITE

I have been looking at a book about studying. It goes into great detail about how you should set aside a room that is reserved for your books and files and in which you quietly gather your thoughts and do your work. Who can afford this sort of extra-room-luxury? Most of us are struggling to find space in the houses that we already have.

My advice is simply this. Find out how you work best. Then, as long as it continues to work, work in that way. I, for example, sit in a corner of the dining room, tapping away at the keys of my computer while, in the adjoining living room, my family sit and watch TV, shout at each other and do all the things that families always do. A large dog and two cats sometimes come and worry me but, generally, I am left alone. If I want to, I can get up and wander into the kitchen to make coffee. Sometimes it is made for me. I can also get up and go and watch the ten o'clock news when it comes on. It is not a good idea to sit in front of a computer screen for hours on end. Watching another screen at least gets you away from the smaller one for a few minutes. Also, it allows you to stretch and it saves you from getting repetitive strain injury from prolonged periods at the keyboard.

I have a pile of books on the floor next to me that I use while I am writing. At the end of a session (if I am in the right mood), I put them all away in bookshelves. Otherwise, I am almost ashamed to write, they stay where they are, until I move them another day or someone else clears them away.

This is the way that I work. It may not suit you. I find that I don't particularly like the cloistered life and don't work well in quiet places. On the other hand, I am not someone who works with the radio or Walkman. Instead, I prefer a fairly 'normal' domestic background. It tends to help me keep my feet on the ground and I hope that this means that my writing is more straightforward. All this applies to **any** sort of writing project. I adopt the same style of working if I am writing up a research report and if I am writing a short article or a book. As I say, it works for me. What works for you? Consider the following places to work. Which would be ideal for you?

- in a quiet office of your own;
- in a public library;
- in the living room with the television on;
- in your bedroom;
- outside;
- in a hotel room;
- in an office at work.

Now consider **where you actually work**. I suspect that most of us have to compromise to some degree about our writing environment. Could you make yours better? By way of example the American writer, William Strong, describes how he works at making initial drafts of written work:

> For me, drafting often works in places like McDonald's where nobody hassles you, the coffee refills are free, and there's a low level of background noise. I prefer pens with laserlike tips. I have an aversion to slick, clay-coated paper and a fondness for cheap note pads, especially soft yellow ones. How about you? (Strong, 1991)

BASIC EQUIPMENT

Certain basic things do seem to count as essentials. While the description above may sound a little rough and ready, my corner of the dinning room is fairly well equipped. I consider that the following are essentials:

- a desk or table
- a computer
- a supply of lined pads

- a supply of computer paper: either continuous (if you use a dot matrix printer) or single sheets (if you use a bubble jet or laser)
- a pot containing plenty of pens and pencils (I find I have to buy new supplies of these regularly as my family help themselves fairly freely. I am also aware that it took me months to find the right sort of pot to put them in. I finally tracked it down in Brittany.)
- a ruler, compass and other drawing implements (for drawing diagrams – if you use a computer well, you may be able to use it for your diagrams)
- bookshelves
- a filing cabinet (by no means essential to everyone but important if you have a tidy mind and like a tidy home)
- Sellotape on a heavy dispenser
- a stapler and a large supply of staples
- paperclips (but keep these away from your printer and from your computer keyboard)
- a clipboard for holding papers while you type at the keyboard
- a disk box for your floppy disks (It cannot be stated too clearly that you **must** backup your computer work as you go. Hard disks in computers fail. If they fail and you have not backed up your work, you have lost it.)
- sticky post-it pads (These are vital for jotting down notes and for keeping a running tally of the number of words that you have written if you are working on a larger project. I like to write a new one at the end of each working session and to leave the old ones in place. In this way, the sheer volume of post-its tells me how near I am to finishing the project.)
- a comfortable chair (Some of the older How To Study books describe the importance of a stoic approach to seating. I would sit in an armchair to work if I could fit one into my work setting. Be comfortable as you work. I can find no place for a straight-backed chair. If you need to be kept awake while you work, you have probably been working too long anyway.)

If you intend to carry on writing, you will have to think carefully about bookshelves. We have about five large bookcases in our house and all of them are full. As a result, we have books piled up everywhere. Sod's law dictates that the book you want is never one that is in a bookshelf. Also, such an arrangement does not endear you to libraries. It is always library books that fall down the backs of piles or lie, spine facing away, at the bottom of a pile of other books. Try to keep library books in their own pile. In this way, you know where to find them and always have them to hand when the reminder notices start coming through the letter box.

Also, spend some time in choosing the desk and chair that you will sit at as you work. There is a variety of purpose-built computer tables available if you are going to work with a computer (and I hope that you are, if you are serious about writing). Such tables can be bulky affairs or they can be economic of space to the point were each item of your equipment is piled one on top of the other in a tidy, if not particularly aesthetically pleasing, tower.

Remember that you have to **live** with the furniture that you buy. While it should be functional, I believe that you should also feel comfortable at it. Be particularly wary of computer desks that have pull-out keyboard holders. In my experience, these tend to be set at a very low level. If you are happy to sit in a low chair, buy one. If not, look for something else. Make sure that you seat is comfortable. Some books about writing tend to take a Spartan approach to seating and suggest that the best work can only be done in a straight-backed chair. The chair that is best for you is one that you are comfortable in. Swivel chairs are widely available but tend not to be very supportive of the back. Some favour 'posture' seating that encourages you to 'kneel' in front of your working surface. These are better for your back and shoulders but try one out before you buy one. Not everyone can cope with sitting in a kneeling position for very long.

There is one other piece of equipment that may be useful, depending on the way you write, and that is a dictaphone. Clearly, they were designed for use by those who do not use computers themselves but who have someone else type out their work. They are, though, very useful for make notes and writing memos on the move. Ideas for essays, papers and articles can all be 'jotted down' by simply speaking into a dictaphone. They take a little getting used to and not everyone can make the shift from writing on paper or on a computer to speaking into a dictaphone. They are, however, remarkable cheap and many are now 'voice-activated': they turn themselves on when you speak into them.

Those who **do** have other people who can type up their work may want to use a dictaphone for writing substantial documents. It is possible to dictate the whole of an essay, project, article or even a book. This is **definitely** not everyone's favourite way of working and to do it properly takes a lot of new learning. Dictation was not, for instance, P. G. Wodehouse's preferred way of working. Although he was writing of the problems of dictating to another person, the problem that he describes, below, applies just as much to dictating into a machine:

Not that I ever thought of dictating [this book] to a stenographer. How anybody can compose a story by word of mouth, face to face with a bored looking secretary with a notebook is more than I can imagine. Yet many authors think nothing of saying 'Ready, Miss Spelvin? Take dictation. Quote No comma Lord Jasper Murgatroyd, comma close quote said no better make it hissed Evangeline comma quote I would not marry you if you were the last man on earth close quote period Quote Well comma, I'm not that last man on earth comma so the point does not arise comma close quote replied Lord Jasper comma twirling his moustache cynically period. And so the long day wore on.'

If I started to do that sort of thing I should be feeling all the time that the girl was saying to herself as she took it down, 'Well comma this beats me period How comma with homes for the feeble minded touting for customers on every side comma has a fathead like this Wodehouse succeeded in remaining at large all these years mark of interrogation.' (Wodehouse, 1934)

It isn't, of course, quite as complicated as this but you do have to learn to cast sentences and then to **say** 'full stop' at the end of each of them. Once learned, the process works quite well.

THE RHYTHM OF WRITING

Just as there are no hard and fast rules about environment, nor are there such rules about the way in which you work. I tend to write best of all late at night. I do not enjoy writing in the morning, so I tend to avoid it. But I am not too sensitive to all this. If I have to write to a deadline, I write at any time of the day.

On the other hand, try to establish a rhythm to your work. It is often a good idea to get warmed up a little by doing various 'domestic' tasks before you settle down to real writing. You can, for instance, back up some files from your hard disk to floppies. You can sort out your reference cards on your files. Do treat this as 'warming up', though and not as work itself. The real work starts when you begin to write. If you have a block of some sort, type **anything** onto the screen to get you started. Alternatively, write the word 'the' at the top of the screen and you will have started. Don't feel that you have to write consecutively. I have explained, elsewhere in this book, that – in longer projects – it is often best to start with a chapter or a section that you will enjoy writing and to leave the trickier parts until you have really got into your stride.

If you can, write every day. Don't be a slave to this rule and if you cannot stand the thought of writing on a particular day, don't worry. You are unlikely to lose the ability to write. I am frequently surprised by how many writers complicate the writing process by setting up all sorts of apparent 'rules' about writing. There are no rules. Find out what suits you best and stick to it. When it stops working, change what you do. If this is a rule, it is an important one. Keep working while what you do is effective. When it ceases to be effective, do something else. It is a basic precept in psychotherapy that the last thing a neurotic person wants to do is to change. They want their symptoms to go away but they do not want to change themselves. Some writers and academics are like this. They want to become better writers but stick, stolidly, to one style of working. Try new things. Do it differently. Then, when it begins to fall into place, stick to the process. The film director, the late Derek Jarman once wrote that 'if you are not a perfectionist, you can get a lot done'. I have found this to be a particularly useful aphorism. You don't have to be a perfectionist. Do the best you can and then accept what you have done. Do not aim at perfection: life is far too short.

Buying a computer 3

The point of this chapter is to identify some of the things that you will need to bear in mind if you are thinking of buying a computer to write with. And I would consider it. There is still a lot of fear surrounding computers. Those who are not frightened by them sometimes take a superstitious view: 'I couldn't write straight into one' or 'It's not the same as writing on a pad of paper'. Of course it's not. It's much better. The big plus about writing with a computer is that you never have to **rewrite**. With a computer, you can bash out your draft, in any form you like. Then you can go slowly through the rushed draft and rescue the best bits. You can change a few words here, move a paragraph there. What you never have to do is start again, with a blank page, and write the whole thing again. That seems, to me, to be a considerable advantage.

Perhaps you take the view that you are too old to take up computing. Certainly, younger people work almost automatically with them. My teenage son taught me almost all I know about computers and computing. I have used a computer to write most of my books and papers and also used one to write course brochures, handouts, adverts, letters and so forth. I keep all my bibliographic references on a computer and I can quickly fish out exactly the reference I need, as I am writing. That means that I no longer have to filter through boxes of cards. A considerable time-saver.

I am still surprised by what computers can do and how much time and effort they can save in the writing process. So don't skip this chapter if you don't have a computer. Don't skip it if you do: there will be things here that you can use. For buying a computer for writing is slightly different to buying a computer as a games machine or as a general-purpose household gadget.

Incidentally, it is not really necessary to know how a computer works in order to use one. I find it useful to think of them as the behavioural psychologists used to think of people. They tended to talk about the 'black box' approach to people: there were inputs and outputs and in between was the 'black box' – the person. So it is with computers.

Computer people sometimes talk of the GIGO principle: garbage in equals garbage out. In practical terms, for you and me, this means that the output from a computer is only as good as the input. Inputs occur through the keyboard and output appears on the screen or is printed. All most of us need to know is that we use the keyboard to make input, we can read what we write at the keyboard on the screen. We can print out what we have written with a printer and we can store our work on one of two main media: floppy disks or hard disks.

The floppy varieties are the ones that are transportable and are usually 3.5 in in size. Hard disks are housed in the computer itself. The smaller hard disks tend to start at 80 mb (megabytes) and go up to gigabyte capacity. An 80 mb hard disk can hold the equivalent of more than 80 3.5 in floppies. At the time of writing, an average hard disk is about 500 mb.

WHAT SORT OF COMPUTER?

Computers come in various shapes and sizes. While IBM set the standard for today's basic personal computer, various 'clones' have been produced by a wide range of companies. It is possible to shop around and to find real bargains in the computer world. One way to do this is to buy one or more of the various monthly computer magazines, if you can pluck up the courage to wade through the sea of middle-aged men and teenage boys in your local W. H. Smith's. The next three sections describe the basic configurations.

It is pointless writing about the finer details of computer chips and sizes. The computer production world is in a constant state of flux. Larger capacity, more compact and cheaper machines seem to be marketed almost every month. What is 'standard' at the time of writing this book is almost certain to be out of date by the time the book is published. Only basic guidelines will be attempted here. As I have suggested above, this is a book about writing and not about computers. The magazines will teach you what you need to know about the innards and keep you up to date.

THE BASIC DESKTOP MODEL

Once, almost all computers were of the desktop variety. These are the sort that sit on your desk and which, if you are lucky, some people will admire. Others, of course, will recoil in horror for some people are still frightened by computers and worry about breaking them. There is, it turns out, little to break with a computer. You are unlikely to do any lasting damage unless you use a sledge-hammer.

The components of a basic, desktop computer are these:

- **The computer itself** An oblong block containing the central processing unit (CPU), the hard disk and the floppy disk drives and various other bits and pieces that drive the whole unit.
- **The keyboard** Nearly always laid out in the traditional, typewriter mode (with a QWERTY keyboard layout). These are now available in various shapes and sizes and some are designed to sit at odd angles to help in the prevention of repetitive strain injury.
- **The mouse** This is an instrument, with two or three buttons, attached by wire to the computer. It allows you to press various on-screen buttons that set off certain functions of the computer. Some notebook computers have a built in, upside down mouse, known as a trackerball, whereas other notebooks use a small joystick in the middle of the keyboard for the same set of functions.
- **The visual display unit (VDU): the screen** These come in a range of different degrees of picture resolution and most, these days, have a coloured screen. It is possible, however, to pick up some real bargains in black and white (or amber) screens. In the end, though, most people are going to prefer working with a colour screen.

This is the traditional computer layout and what most people probably think of when they think of a computer. The advantages of this sort of layout are these:

- the keyboard is full size and allows you to work as you would with a type-writer;
- the screen is a full size one and lets you see your work as you write, without too much eye strain;
- the hard-disk capacity of such machines is nearly always potentially bigger than is the case with portable computers.

If you are going to buy a computer, want a bargain and have the room, buy a desktop computer – or, if you can afford it, buy a really well specified, colour notebook and use it as your all-round machine.

THE LAPTOP

The laptop is one of three sorts of portable computer. They are fairly large and fairly heavy machines which open up like briefcases to reveal a keyboard and screen. They can have fairly large hard disks and the screen resolution of such machines is improving all the time. 'Portable' is a relative term. If you do not mind the weight and only want a fairly small hard disk, you can pick up some real bargains. Laptops have been largely replaced by **notebook** computers (described below) and can be picked up very cheaply in some of the computer stores that specialize in less-than-state-of-the-art computers.

THE NOTEBOOK

The notebook computer is smaller and lighter than the laptop. It is very light (about 5 lbs, total weight). It is usually about the size of an A4 pad of paper and contains a keyboard, screen, hard and floppy disk drives. These are usually more expensive than laptops but much more portable. You can fit one inside a briefcase. Not so robust as laptops, some people find the keyboard more cramped than their larger cousins. They are the real solution to computing on the move and it is quite possible to carry with you a half-written research report, the whole manuscript of a book, yards of notes and all of your bibliographic references. If you can afford one, think about buying one of these as a second computer. If you really like them, think about one as your **only** computer. These days, the keyboards and screens are improving all the time.

On the other hand, some people find that notebook computers are too small and light. It is not as simple as it looks to balance on your knee: they tend to fall over backwards. Also, the size and weight of them tend to limit the clarity and visibility of the screen. As I have noted throughout this chapter, things are changing all the time. It seems likely that notebook screens will improve dramatically and quickly.

There is yet another sub-set of the notebook computer known as the 'subnotebook'. This is slightly smaller than the notebook computer but very much lighter. Oddly enough, the subnotebook has not sold all that well at the time of writing. It seems that people still want something a little substantial when they buy a computer.

THE PALMTOP

The palmtop computer is the smallest of all. Often weighing less than a pound, it really is a miniature machine. It has a tiny keyboard and screen, runs on batteries and can be carried in a pocket. It is, however, a **real** computer. It usually has built in programs that include a word processor, a spreadsheet, a diary and a calculator. The palmtop is often sold as a 'personal information manager' and is used as a replacement for a diary. It can be used for writing of all sorts, from note-writing to the production of papers and articles. Its great advantage is that it is highly portable and can be used almost anyway. Its great disadvantage is that the keyboard is so small that it does not suit some users.

Portable computers can be stolen. Their portability means that they can easily be removed by other people and it is quite possible to leave them at stations or airports if you are not used to travelling with them. If you **do** find yourself travelling with a computer (and it can make sense if you take writing seriously but also have to travel), then you need to consider **insurance** for it. Classe (1995) offers the following pointers for consideration when looking for insurance for portable computers:

- Does your present insurance cover you for habitual use of notebook computers outside the office?
- Are you covered if you take the computer overseas?
- Watch out for exclusion clauses in insurance policies. You may not be covered if you leave a portable in an unattended car – even if it is in the boot. Cover in hotel rooms may depend on the security classification of thehotel. You may not be covered in someone else's office or if you lend your computer to anyone.
- Check excesses on claims. An excess of £250 could end up costing you as much as the repair.

Perhaps most important of all, however, you **must** make backups of all of the data files on a portable. While this rule applies to all computers and computing, it applies even more to portable ones. If your portable computer is stolen, it is unlikely that you will get your essays, dissertation or articles back. If you have access to your computer and you know that you have work on it that is not backed up, get up and back it up now! It is as serious as that.

PRINTERS

There are now three main sorts of printers:

- dot matrix
- ink jet
- laser

Dot matrix printers work by using a series of between 9 and 36 pins which put tiny blobs of ink onto the paper in the shape of characters. They tend to be noisy and slow and can rarely match the speed of the other two sorts. They are, once you set them up correctly (see lament below), easy to operate, cheap to run and generally efficient.

Ink jet printers work by spraying fine bursts of ink onto the page. Sometimes these are bubbles of ink and those printers have been called 'bubble jet printers', but the term 'ink jet printers' is now generally applied to both types. Both are almost silent, fairly speedy, cheaper to operate than laser printers and cheaper to buy. They have been called the poor person's laser printer. Their only real drawback is that one replaceable cartridge of ink for the ink jet does not print very many pages. This can mean that you pay out quite a lot for new ones and that you may have to break longer printing sessions into small parts. Some companies sell equipment that allows you to replace the ink in the cartridges. These can cut down the cost of using these printers considerably. At the time of writing, ink jet printers offer the best, all-round value for money. They are only slightly more expensive than dot matrix printers but offer considerably higher quality of printout.

Ink jet printers are available in a colour option at only a relatively small increase in price. Most writers probably will not need a colour printer but, increasingly, colour work is being used in the production of charts and diagrams and may soon be an integral part of most postgraduate dissertations and theses.

The laser printer is the one to go for if you can afford it. They work in a similar way to photocopiers and are very quick, easy to use and almost silent in operation. They produce very high quality printout and the end-product looks more like a printed page than the typewritten page that tends to be produced by a dot matrix printer.

BUYING A COMPUTER FOR WRITING

What computer should you buy? Computer hardware (the keyboard, monitor and computing unit itself) is changing rapidly. It is also dropping in price. Any specific advice about particular models of computer would be out of place. Certain general suggestions may be made. A computer for use in the home, that is not going to age too quickly should fulfil most and perhaps all of the following criteria:

- It should be IBM compatible if it is to be compatible with all Windows programs. IBM set a certain standard for computing equipment at the end of the 1980s. While many computers are 'IBM clones' and while it is not necessary to buy a genuine IBM machine, it is essential that the computer that you buy is fully compatible with IBM machines, if you want to use the sorts of programs described in this book. The other option (which is not discussed here) is the Apple Macintosh. I fully appreciate that many people use Apple Macintoshes and that they are just as good as the IBM-compatible sort (which are also called PCs). It is just that the IBMs and compatible computers are more widely used and that is why this chapter has concentrated on them. In recent years, however, there has also been a third option: the PowerMac – an Apple Macintosh computer that can also work with software made for IBM compatible machines.
- It should have a hard disk. A hard (as opposed to a floppy) disk is capable of storing vast amounts of data. While larger capacity floppy disks are being developed, hard disks currently allow for the storage of 100, 300, 500 mb of data and above. The hard disk also allows you to store all of your programs inside the computer and saves you having to find disks and load up programs from 'outside'. In my experience, it is impossible to overestimate the size of the hard disk that you will need. Faced with 200 mb of space, it is tempting to think that you will never fill it up. Faced with 500 mb you are likely to think it is impossible. I know many writers who have filled 500 mb hard disks and are looking for more space. Get the largest you can afford. Larger hard disks also tend to be faster than smaller ones. These days, Windows programs, themselves, occupy very large amounts of hard disk space. This means that less space will be available for text files if you use a fairly small

hard disk. As a rule, you cannot go wrong buying a very large hard disk.

- It should be expandable. Many computers have 'expansion slots' inside them which allow for upgrading in line with current technological developments. Some of the cheaper and smaller ones do not. It is not necessary to keep changing hardware to keep up with every development. On the other hand, if you do not keep up with some of the **main** developments, you may find that you can no longer find software to work with your computer as it gets older.

- It should have a monitor and keyboard that suit you. On the monitor issue, many feel that a black and white screen is ideal for word-processing. On the other hand, some feel that a colour screen gives them more flexibility. Yet others prefer a large size screen that allow you to see and work on a whole A4 page of print at a time. Obviously, larger screens also cost more and are 'non-standard'. Similarly, the 'feel' of a keyboard is the subject of much debate. Some prefer a keyboard that reminds them of a typewriter and 'clicks' when the keys are pressed. Others prefer a 'deader' keyboard. It is recommended that you try typing on a range of keyboards before you choose yours. This is one of the problems when buying computers through the post. Unless you have had experience of the model that you order, you will not be able to try out the keyboard before you buy. I suspect, though, that the keyboard question is only an issue when you first buy a computer. After a couple of weeks, you get used to the feel of the keyboard and no longer worry about whether or not it 'clicks'. I work on a range of keyboards in my job and I don't find any of them particularly objectionable – and I touch type.

- It should have sufficient RAM (random access memory) to allow you to use modern programs. As computers develop, so the random access memory requirements grow. Until fairly recently, a computer that had 640 kb of memory was thought to be adequate. Then the usual figure was 1 mb. Now it is not uncommon to find machines with 8 mb fitted as standard. If you cannot afford to buy a computer with a lot of RAM fitted as standard, make sure that you can expand the memory at a later date. Like most aspects of computers, the price of RAM is dropping all the time. If you plan to run basic Windows programs, 8 mb is probably the minimum that you should buy. If you intend to use large graphics or statistics packages, you will not regret buying 16 mb of RAM.

WHERE DO I BUY IT?

There are a number of ways of buying a computer. First, though, you need to choose which one you are going to buy. If you already have one and are upgrading, you are likely to know what sort you want. In the end, there is little to choose between the various makes in terms of quality. These days, nearly all computers are of high quality. You will pay extra for the big names. You will also pay extra for on-site maintenance. You may also pay extra for telephone help. In my experience, the last is vital. For some reason, I have never yet been able to make a printer work with a computer, first time.

Talk to people who know about computers before you buy one. Whilst they often have odd favourites and can be a rather quirky crowd, they can usually offer good advice about what to buy. If you know what you want, it is safe and usually much cheaper to buy by mail order. These days, you can ring up with a credit card and the machinery is installed in your home by the end of the week. It will be fully set up and configured by the company and usually you will be able to secure on-site maintenance if anything goes wrong.

If you are not sure what you want, you can have a look at some computers produced by the larger firms in your local electrical supermarket. You will tend to pay more if you buy them in this way and the assistants in such shops do not tend to know very much about computers. They are not there to be computer experts. They are there to sell machines. On the whole, I would avoid buying in this way. You are often better off (literally) going to a dedicated computer shop. These are often away from the high street but sell nothing but computers and computer-related goods. They can offer the same service as the mail order firms and are usually only a little more expensive. My advice would be to buy a cheap computer from one of the Tottenham Court Road (London) computer stores. Use it for about a year and learn all that you can about computers. Then buy the machine that you really want through a mail order firm. The Tottenham Court Road shops sell **real** bargains.

If you become a full-time writer or a part-time one who is registered as a writer for tax purposes, you may be able to **lease** computing equipment. The point about leasing is that you can offset the whole of the cost of the leasing agreement against tax. In effect, your computer is essential business equipment.

ADD-ONS

There is a whole range of other hardware that you can buy to add to your computer. A short list of these includes the following.

- **A modem** This is a card that slots into your computer or a separate item that plugs into it. A modem makes use of telephone lines and allows you to send messages and data to other computer users. You are also able to 'download' computer programs that have been sent down the telephone line. The great thing about a modem, though, is that (with the right software and the right connection) it will allow you access to the Internet. This is a worldwide 'network of networks' which will enable you to obtain information about all sorts of things from anywhere in the world. At one level, it is like a huge, international library. Many people, though, use it for e-mail (electronic mail) – a system that allows you to send messages, letters, reports, pictures and computer files to other people anywhere in the world.
- **A back-up system** You must back up the data that you store on your hard disk. Most people, using small hard disks, back up their work to floppy

disks. If you have a larger one, you may want to invest in a 'tape streamer'. This is a small machine, rather like a tape recorder that allows you to duplicate everything that is on your hard disk. This sort of add-on becomes more important with larger hard disks. Remember, though, that you only have to back up your data disks. Your programs are already 'backed up' in that you have them on floppy disks, separate to your hard disk.

- **More disk space**   If your hard disk gets filled up (and they do get filled up quite quickly) then you can simply slot in a hard card. This is a hard disk on a card that fits in one of the expansion slots inside your computer.

- **CD-ROM** (Compact-disc, Read Only Memory)   The CD-ROM add-on uses compact disc to store massive amounts of data. That data can only be read from the discs. You cannot (at the moment) write to a compact disc. Thus it is possible to review the contents of the disc and to call up the sections that you want into your computer. Compact discs are available that list bibliographical references, encyclopaedias and even the complete works of Shakespeare. Further details of some of the CD-ROMS available and useful to the writer are detailed below.

- **A scanner**   This allows you to transfer images and text from the printed page into the computer. To transfer text, you need special software (Optical Character Recognition software). Don't assume that all scanners are sold with this software and make sure that the scanner you buy will be able to make use of it. A scanner will enable you to transfer typed notes straight from the page into your computer. Don't expect (at the moment) that it will allow you to transfer all your handwritten notes into a format that can be edited in a word processor. The technology involved in recognizing handwriting is still in the elementary stage.

- **A voice recognition system**   Talk to your computer! A voice recognition system allows you to dictate into your computer and have the computer produce your words on the screen. First, though, you have to 'teach' the computer about the way that you speak and about the words that you use through a fairly lengthy setting up process. Also, don't expect that you can simply talk at a normal speed, in a normal tone and have the computer produce your ideas in a perfect format. At the moment, voice recognition systems are fairly primitive. You have to speak very clearly and fairly slowly and the production of mistakes is fairly high. Only use such a system if you really cannot use a keyboard or if you have money and time to burn – voice recognition systems are expensive and take a long time to set up and use.

THE INTERNET

The Internet, Cyberspace, the information superhighway: these are all terms that students, managers and clinicians are going to meet in the next few weeks, months and years. They refer to a huge 'network of networks' – a world-wide linking up of computers and computer networks.

It is likely that the Internet is going to change the way many people handle and process information. Just a brief look at the things you can do with the Internet can give a clue to how managers, educators and students will be able to use the system. First, they will have access to huge amounts of information – from papers, books and files. Second, they will be able to make contact with lots of like-minded people who share their research, management or clinical interests. They will be able to search for publications, contact specialists in other countries and even set up international 'real time' conferences.

So to access the Internet what do you need? A computer, a modem and a bridge into a computer network. Most colleges and university departments run a networked computer system and many will allow their staff to plug into this network. After that, it is a question of learning how to negotiate your way around the Internet. This is where some reading matter can help.

There are two excellent introductory guides to the Internet. *The Internet for Dummies* by Levine and Baroudi (1993) offers a humorous and easy to digest account of all aspects of setting up an Internet link and negotiating your way around it. I doubt that it will suit the real beginner. It is likely to be more useful to someone who knows a little about computers and a little about the jargon that is used. On the other hand, it doesn't assume very much and most people who are totally new to the Internet will find this a useful starting point.

A different approach is taken in *How the Internet Works* by John Eddings (1994). This is a beautifully prepared book and offers both text and cleverly devised illustrations. It is almost a 'picture-book' account of how the Internet works. There is not a lot of text for your money but the mixture of text and graphics is likely to make learning a lot easier.

Once you have grasped the basics of the Internet, you will need to know where to start looking for information. What is needed is some sort of 'telephone directory': a listing of who's who in the Internet world. There are two particularly useful books on this issue. The first is Hahn and Stout's *The Internet Yellow Pages* (1994) – which is just that: a listing of contacts under a huge range of subject headings. This approach is bound to develop over the years and no doubt soon every town will have its 'Internet Pages'. Until then, Hahn and Stout's book fills an important gap.

Similarly, Que Corporation's *The Internet Resource: Quick Reference* (1994) is another form of listing of contacts. This one is arranged alphabetically rather than by subject matter. If you know the specific area of information that you are looking for, this book will be particularly useful. Together, *The Internet Yellow Pages* and *The Internet Resource* make a valuable pair of resource books that will be essential reference books for any Internet user.

SOFTWARE

Your computer, on its own, will be of no use to you. You will have to have programs to run on it. These are discussed in the next chapter. Make sure, though, that you have an 'operating system' already on your hard disk when you buy your machine. An operating system is the basic software that allows your computer to read programs. Unfortunately (and it seems overcomplicated to my simple mind) you cannot just run programs direct. First, you have to have a skeleton system working away in the background. At the moment, for personal computers, there are two common operating systems. One is called Disk Operating System (**DOS**) the other is called **Windows**. (Note that the Apple-Mac has its own operating system that is not directly compatible with those of the IBM-compatibles.)

DOS relies on the user's being familiar with certain words to make the programs come alive ('commands') and is thus know as a command-driven system. Windows lets you use a mouse to drag the cursor to symbols and icons on the screen in order to start and work with programs. Which you prefer is, to some degree, a matter of taste. It is, however, more complicated than that and I recommend that you talk to your local supplier about the other differences between the two systems. There are other operating systems but it seems that DOS, Windows and variants on these are likely to be the most frequently used systems for the near future.

In future, **Microsoft**, the makers of Windows, plan to name new editions of the program according to the year in which they are produced. (Thus the version that came out in 1995 is known as Windows 95.) Whether or not this means that a new version will be produced every year remains to be seen. It is also likely that all Microsoft programs running under Windows will be revised every year in line with these revisions of Windows, itself.

Once an operating system has been installed on your machine, you can forget it. It fires up when you switch on and it works away in the background without your having to think very much about it. If you want to and if you like that sort of thing, you can also spend a lifetime learning all about the ins and outs of your operating system. It is probably better to spend the time **writing** on the computer.

WORD PROCESSORS

The most important computer program for the writer is the word processor. Word processors for the personal computer come in many shapes and sizes. As a minimum, you want one that can perform the following functions:

- count words;
- spell-check;
- move text around;
- set margins;
- show text on the screen in roughly the same format as you will see it on the printed page. If you use some word processors running under Windows,

you will see the text almost exactly as it appears on paper. This is called WYSIWYG – What You See Is What You Get.

Also, you want a word processor that is easy to use. Most take a little time to learn and some of the larger ones have huge numbers of functions. In my experience, people tend to think that they will not want all the extra functions. For everyday use, this is true. There comes a time, though, when you **will** use some of the more esoteric functions. Examples of these other functions include:

- the ability to sort lines or paragraphs of text, alphabetically or by number;
- the ability to 'search and replace': searching for strings of characters and replacing them;
- the ability to use 'bullets' such as the ones in this list;
- the ability to work with more than one document at once;
- the ability to create indexes;
- the ability to work with very long textual documents;
- the ability to change font sizes;
- the ability to create 'macros': keyboard short cuts that allow you to access some of the more complicated aspects of the word-processing program;
- the use of a thesaurus for checking and changing words;
- the use of a **bolding** facility that prints blacker characters;
- the ability to import graphical images;
- the ability to import spreadsheet tables;
- the ability to apply pre-set 'styles' to a document to make sure that it is laid out consistently.

The list can go on. Only the larger commercial word-processing programs are likely to contain all of these functions. For me, the important things in considering what word processor to buy are these:

- ease of use;
- range of functions.

What follows is a brief review of some of the better known word-processing packages. The important thing is to find the package that you are most comfortable with. Most word-processor users tend to think that the one that they use is the best. I admit to being a Word for Windows fan and I am constantly surprised at what it can do. Four years later, I am still learning some of its more rarely used functions but when I do need them, I usually find that they are easy to use. There seems to be a critical period, in learning to use a word processor. Somehow, you need to spend time getting the hang of the 'whole' of the program. Once you have this overall feel for how the program operates, you seem to relax and are able to take a more leisurely approach to some of the finer details.

The particular virtue of Windows programs is that they all look fairly similar on the screen. This means that switching from one program to another is much easier than it used to be. If you can learn **one** Windows program, you can easily learn others. Also, it is easy to transfer files across from one word processor to another. Most of the main Windows word processors have the facility for saving a file in the format of another. This is particularly useful if you are working on a project with another person who is using a different word processor.

WordPerfect

In the DOS field, at the time of writing, WordPerfect is still the world's best selling word-processing program. It seems likely to remain the market leader as software development has moved away from DOS in recent years to concentrate on Windows programs. WordPerfect has a huge range of features that will satisfy anyone who has to produce text. All of the functions can be accessed either through the 'function' keys (F1–F12) or through a series of pull-down menus. You can also use a mouse with it. The program can be personalized and you can modify the keyboard to suit your own style of working.

Some people have been critical of the fact that WordPerfect uses the function keys. This can be a drawback to touch typists who have to take their fingers off the keyboard to reach those keys. On the other hand, like most other mainstream word processors, WordPerfect can be customized, extensively, to suit the individual user. The program is expensive and regular updates are offered which the user has to decide whether or not to buy. WordPerfect is available both in a DOS and a Windows version. The Windows version came on the scene rather later than did Word for Windows and has lagged behind ever since.

Word for Windows

Word for Windows is a fully featured word-processing package and one that is ideal for writers. Apart from all the usual word-processing features that we will explore in the next chapter, Word for Windows allows you to work with multiple documents. You might, for example, want to work with a variety of versions of an essay or an article and the program allows you to switch, quickly, between the various versions. The program also has a very versatile 'undo' feature. As you work at polishing your essay or report, you may find that you don't like the last series of 'edits' that you made. Using the undo feature, you can quickly 'take off' the editing (and, just as easily, 'put back' the editing).

The program is very easy to customize, according to how you work. You can set up the usual range of 'macros' (or short cuts). You can also develop 'button bars' – sets of buttons that sit at the top of the screen that allow you to perform certain functions quickly. On the button bar on the version I am using to write these words, for example, I have buttons to do the following:

- set up the sub heading styles;
- count the words in a whole document;

- select all of the text in a document (this is useful if you want to make 'global' changes to a document);
- find and replace selections of text
- call up a copy of my CV;
- insert the full name and 'path' of a document as a footnote on every page;
- call up the file that contains the manuscript of this book (when the book is finished and the publishers are happy with the manuscript, this button will be taken off the button bar).

WordPerfect for Windows

WordPerfect for Windows is another fully featured word processor and contains many of the features that can be found in Word for Windows. It does, however, have quite a different 'feel' to Word and many of the functions work in different ways. Like most Windows word processors, however, it has the familiar pull-down menus at the top of the screen and rows of buttons that can be customized. It also has an excellent file-handling system that allows you to preview files before you open them. This is particularly useful if you are not sure of the **name** that you gave to a file and want to have a quick look at the file in question before you open it up on the screen.

One important point should be borne in mind for the person who plans to switch from WordPerfect for DOS to WordPerfect for Windows. The two programs, although written by the same company are very different. It cannot be assumed that the seasoned WordPerfect 5.1 or 6.0 user will find the Windows version 'intuitive' to use. He or she will need to work at 'relearning' the new program. The effort, however, is worth it as Windows programs are always easier to use than DOS ones, once the initial learning curve has been mastered.

There are lots of other word-processing packages that you may want to explore. A shortlist of them includes:

- Ami Pro
- WordStar for Windows
- LetterPerfect
- Locoscript PC

OTHER PROGRAMS FOR THE WRITER

The suite of programs

There are a number of packages on the market that supply you with a whole range of programs, together. These are known as **suites** and usually contain and fully featured word processor, a spreadsheet, a database and a graphics program. At the moment, the 'big three' packages are Microsoft Office, Novell Office and Lotus SmartSuite. This is an ideal way to buy a number of important programs together. Buying a suite is always cheaper than buying the individual programs separately and the companies that make these suites often offer special prices to induce people to change from one company's programs to another. If you are a WordPerfect user, for example, you will probably be able to 'cross platforms' to Microsoft Office for a remarkably cheap price.

The point, obviously, is that you need to know that you are going to **use** the other programs, before you buy a suite. Spreadsheets are ideal if you are going to be working with numbers – a spreadsheet is a huge matrix of 'rows and columns' and it allows you to manipulate figures in all sorts of ways. Databases are likely to be useful to most writers and can be used to store all sorts of structured information, from bibliographical references to names and addresses. Graphics programs are also useful to the technical writer. While most word processors allow you to produce bar chats, histograms and graphs, dedicated graphics programs usually allow you to do these things better. If you want to illustrate your work in other ways, too, you will make use of a graphics package.

The alternative to the suite is the **integrated package**. Integrated packages are programs that contain features of word processors, spreadsheets, databases and graphics programs all in the one program. Whereas a suite is a **set** of discrete programs (which can usually work together), the integrated package is **one** program containing 'cut down' aspects of the larger programs. Examples of integrated packages include Microsoft Works and Claris Works. Most integrated packages have 'Works' in their titles.

Edmunds (1995) offers the following buyer's checklist for the person who is considering buying a suite of programs or an integrated package:

- If you are considering buying more than one mainstream application from the same publisher you should probably consider buying the suite.
- Integrated packages require less computer resources than software suites but include fewer features. Check that any features you require are included.
- If you expect to make a lot of use of one particular application in the integrated package, say a word processor, you will be better off buying the full version rather than relying on a reduced feature set.
- Special suite prices are available from all vendors when upgrading from a competitive or earlier product.
- Most integrated Windows packages will operate adequately on a 20 mHz 386SX with 4 mb RAM and a 40 mb hard disk.
- If your machine is less than a 25 mHz 486SX with 8 mb RAM and a 200 mb hard disk, you will not be able to make full use of a software suite. A 66 mHz 486DX2 and 16 mb RAM is recommended.
- At under £100 integrated packages are exceptional value but skimping on software if users really need the feature sets of complete applications may not pay off in the long term.

Oxford Writer's Shelf and other Oxford programs

Anyone who has to write a report, a paper or a book needs access to the tools of writing: a dictionary, a thesaurus, an encyclopaedia and, perhaps, some books of quotations. Until now, the usual route to these tools has been through books. Now, they are available as software programs.

Oxford University Press has published a range of their best reference works as Windows programs. The first collection – **Oxford Writer's Shelf** – was previously available as a DOS program. The new version is both easier to use and contains more works.

Oxford Writer's Shelf is a package that brings together the following reference texts: *The Oxford Dictionary for Writers and Editors, The Oxford Guide to English Usage, The Pocket Oxford Dictionary, Minidictionary of Quotations* and *The Macmillan Compact Encyclopaedia*. In this way, key works are available at the touch of the mouse.

All, some or one of the volumes can be loaded onto your hard disk and access is via the usual Windows icons. Installation from floppy disks is a painless procedure and after that – as with any Windows programs – the Oxford 'books' can be popped up over any other program that you are working with. Thus you can check a meaning or consult the encyclopaedia as you are working on your paper or report. Each title in the Shelf allows you to consult the table of contents, browse through the entries, search for a keyword, look up cross-references and copy text into your own documents via the clipboard.

You can customize the Shelf in various ways. You can, for example, decide which book is 'opened' by default when you fire up the program. I found it most useful to have the dictionary as the default book. This meant that a new dimension was added to an already fully featured word processor. While most modern word processors have spell-checking and thesaurus facilities, none that I know of also contain a dictionary. The addition is very welcome.

At first I thought the idea of an 'on-line' dictionary and encyclopaedia was overkill. It seemed easier to reach for a 'real' dictionary. After a few days, however, it became clear that having the works to hand without moving away from the computer was a real advantage. While laziness might stop you from checking a word if the dictionary was in another room, with the book as an integral part of the computer, there was no excuse!

Anyone who needs to write formal reports will appreciate the advice contained in *The Oxford Dictionary for Writers and Editors* and the whole suite of books will be of value to those who write professionally or for courses. The Windows version of the Shelf has been very well realized. It is easy to use, dramatically fast and very useful.

Other 'Shelves' are available as part of the series. OUP also publish *The Oxford Business Shelf* and *The Oxford Language Shelf*.

Two other Oxford publications are also of considerable interest. Both form part of another set of integrated programs. First, *The Concise Oxford Dictionary* is available as a Windows program. It works in a similar way to the Shelf programs and offers immediate access to the new and best-selling 8th edition of this acclaimed dictionary. Clearly, this is a more comprehensive work than the *Pocket Oxford Dictionary* and if your needs are likely to stop at a good dictionary, this is probably the one to go for. *The Concise Oxford Dictionary* can be made to integrate seamlessly with Microsoft's Word for Windows – probably the best selling Windows word processor. The fact that you can switch straight into the dictionary from Word for Windows adds more value to the Oxford product.

Also available and uniform with *The Concise Oxford Dictionary* is *The Oxford Dictionary of Quotations and Modern Quotations*. All the things that you can do with the Shelf programs you can do with these programs. That means that you can import quotations directly out of the program and into your report, essay or book.

These are impressive programs that have been well designed and executed. They will be of immense value to anyone who has to write. My only complaint is that the Shelf programs cannot be automatically integrated with the *COD* and the *Dictionary of Quotations*. Perhaps in future editions of the programs, it will be possible to put *The Concise Oxford Dictionary* on the same 'shelf' as *The Oxford Guide to English Usage* and click one icon to bring up all the books in the two series.

All of the programs are attractively produced. The boxes containing the disks and manuals can even sit on **real** shelves and look like **real** books. On the computer, the books soon become essential tools in the process of producing words.

EndNote Plus

EndNote Plus is a program designed for working with bibliographical references and is ideal for the writer who works with a DOS-based word processor. What does it do? Talking through a typical application of the program is probably the best way of describing how EndNote Plus works in practice.

You can run the program in various ways. First, it can be run on its own as a free standing reference's database program. Then, it can be used as a 'terminate and stay resident' (TSR) program that can be popped up over WordPerfect. Many people are likely to find this a useful way of working with it. Finally, it can be run through Windows and alongside a range of other programs.

This is one way of using it. Imagine that you are working on an essay or a paper in your word processor. You want to support an argument with a reference but you cannot quite remember the particular article or book. You call up EndNote Plus and browse through your reference collection. Finding the right paper, you mark it, press a couple of buttons to transfer the reference to the program's 'clipboard' and then you return to your word processor. You then press another couple of buttons and a note about the reference is pasted straight into your essay.

When you have finished working through your essay or paper in this way – collecting references from EndNote Plus as you work – you then have to think about how the reference list at the end of your paper will be formatted. You may, for example, want to use the Vancouver or the Harvard referencing system (for more about these see pp. 105–109). On the other hand, the journal to which you are submitting your paper may lay down very specific instructions about how to list your references. All of this presents no problem to EndNote Plus. At the end of your paper you simply ask the program to format your reference list in any one of a wide range of referencing styles including all the main 'academic' ones and many of the most common journal styles.

Now imagine another possibility. You send your paper off to the journal but it is not accepted for publication. You modify it a little and then send it off to another. Before you do that, you realize that the new journal requires another style of referencing. Again, this presents no problems. EndNote Plus allows you simply to change all of the references and your final list to suit the requirements of the second journal. In theory you could go on doing this ad nauseam.

EndNote Plus offers an incredible amount of flexibility in storing, sorting, searching and organizing your reference collection. It will also generate ASCII files for transferring information to other programs and will work 'automatically' with Microsoft Word and WordPerfect. It is also fully compatible with EndNote and EndNote Plus on the Apple Macintosh.

Reference collections are both personal and valuable. This program not only helps you to cite references in papers and articles, it also encourages you to build your own reference library. Not only of books and papers but also of computer software and other forms of 'text'. You can do simple and complex searches and build reference collections up to 32 000 entries long. It would make an ideal institutional as well as personal purchase. It comes with a very well-written manual and a large number of pre-set 'forms' for entering your references. If you do not like the ones you find, you can make your own. It is worth spending some time learning to use this program to its limit. It will be time well spent and will quickly be repaid by the time and energy you save when you start using the program as a writing aid.

Norton Utilities

Everyone does it at some point. You press a couple of wrong keys and suddenly the file you are working on disappears forever. You stab wildly at the keyboard. You repeat a series of keystrokes over and over again like a rat in a psychologist's laboratory. Nothing brings your file back. At this point, you may decide that computers are not for you. Or you may burst into tears. You could reach for **Norton Utilities**.

Norton Utilities is a huge package of programs that every serious computer user will find useful. The situation, above, is just one in which Utilities could help. It can rescue deleted files and even deleted disks. As someone who once deleted a complete book chapter I was working on, I only wish that I had had this program three years ago.

Norton Utilities has been around, in various versions, for some years. This latest version offers a highly integrated but easy to use set of utility programs for anyone who wants to use and maintain his or her computer to the utmost. The various elements of the program are drawn together via a menu screen that can be operated either with a mouse or with the keyboard. It is intuitive to use and the program is simple to install. Indeed, the menu system is almost **too** easy to use. Norton Utilities contains some very powerful and (to the novice) potentially dangerous programs. It would not be difficult to find yourself firing up these parts of the programs. So key with care. Some parts of the program are not for the novice.

Here are some of the things that Norton Utilities can do. First, as noted above, it can recover accidentally wiped data. It can also help in those cases where the computer crashes in the middle of a program leaving data scattered around your hard disk. It can also repair damaged data files and this function might be vital if you keep large database or spreadsheet files.

It can also speed up your hard disk. It can give you a very detailed analysis of both your computer and your hard disk. You can then adjust the interleave factor of your hard disk and compress all of the files on it. Over a period of time, the hard disk gets to be 'fragmented'. This means that bits of files are written all over it, in no particular order. Part of the Norton Utilities suite can rearrange your files, 'end to end' or contiguously. This can speed up the functioning of your hard disk quite considerably. As if that were not enough, Norton Utilities also offers you a disk cache. A disk cache stores frequently read data from your hard disk and acts as an extremely fast section of memory. This part of the utilities program is not very easy to set up and I found it was not particularly happy working with my high memory manager. It does seem, however, faster than the caching program that comes with DOS – Smartdrive. You may want to experiment with this.

Therein lies the problem. Norton Utilities might have been made for the compulsive 'fiddler'. It has so many functions – most of which seem interesting – that you can spend hours fine-tuning your computer. I suspect that a whole generation of computer users is evolving. These are people who produce very little from their machines but who always have those machines functioning optimally. Here is one example of the sort of thing that will appeal to fiddlers. On a colour screen, the program allows you to alter the basic screen colour and then the colour of the text that you type onto the screen.

As with most utility programs, Norton Utilities offers an extensive menuing and file management program. It allows you to bypass the DOS prompt and view all of your files in their directories and subdirectories. It also enables you to keep a list of your programs and start them up at the touch of a button; it has an extensive 'help' section that is easy to use and genuinely helpful; and has some of the best documentation I have read. The easy-to-read manual is packed with tips on how to maximize your system. The manuals also teach you a lot about hard disks and hard-disk management.

Clean Sweep

Windows programs are famous for distributing odd files all over your hard disk. **Clean Sweep** is a program that does a small number of things really well. It finds files on your hard disk that you do not use, duplicate files and 'lost' files from programs that have been deleted. It then allows you to remove these programs from the hard disk. In this way, you can free up remarkable large amounts of hard-disk space. There are other 'uninstall' programs on the market and all do much the same sort of thing. This one is easy to use and worth the investment.

Dashboard

Most people who use PCs are changing to Windows as a user interface. The advantages are clear: you can achieve true 'what you see is what you get' effects; you can run more than one program at a time; and because Windows programs mostly use the same screen layout, you can soon learn other programs once you have mastered one.

Windows is not known for its speed. Anything that simplifies and speeds up running time is to be welcomed. **Dashboard** is a very compact, very fast and very useful product. Borrowing the analogy of a car dashboard, it fits into a slim bar the following features: quick-start program icons, access to other program groups, a 'speedo' that monitors your memory usage, a clock, a printer controller and a feature that allows you to switch quickly between applications that you are using.

What is striking about the program is the fact that it can be customized to match the way that you work. If you want access to all your program icons, at all times, then you simply modify Dashboard into a single row of icons running along the bottom or down the side of your screen. If, on the other hand, you want a whole range of indicators and buttons to control all aspects of your computing work, you can have that too. Dashboard can be made to run 'on top' of all other programs, so that it is always visible. It can also be used as a replacement for the Windows Program Manager shell.

The 'minimalist' user will appreciate this level of customization. You can change your computer screen from being a mass of windows and icons to one that contains nothing more than the Dashboard screen. And Dashboard will enable you to launch your programs, keep an eye on your memory resources, print out files by the 'drag and drop' method and watch the time. The overall ffect is to bring together all the power of the Windows approach to computing with none of the fuss. It also offers the **fastest** way of starting and switching programs.

Publisher

In these cost-conscious days, most health care writers have to prepare booklets, reports, flyers and advertisement copy. With a laser printer and a little thought, it is possible to produce good-looking, high-quality text. You need the right software, though.

Publisher is the sort of program for people who were always nervous of desktop publishing programs. In the past, you were normally faced with a blank sheet of paper on the computer screen that you had to try to manipulate. Publisher still offers you that same sheet of paper but it also holds your hand as you work through the process of producing documents (or 'publications' as Microsoft would like you to call them).

On starting Publisher, you are invited to choose an approach to working. If you know what you are doing, you can go straight for the 'blank sheet' approach. Or you could use a **template**. Templates offer you pre-set layouts for a considerable range of business documents. One, for example, will help you to do a layout for a brochure to publicize your organization. Others will enable you to design posters, flyers, fax cover sheets and so on. All you do is select the template and then fill in the blanks. This is the 'intermediate' starting position – perhaps for the person who has **some** experience of working with a desktop publishing program, but not very much.

The ultimate in help, though, comes from **Page Wizards**. These are a particularly attractive and easy way of working. The Wizard asks you to select a particular type of document and then asks you a series of questions about that document. It asks you, for example, to select the 'style' of your new creation. It then asks you for some heading text and various questions about how you would like pictures and/or text to be laid out. Finally, you just have to sit back and watch the Wizard create your document for you. This is good on a number of counts. First, it is interesting to see your document being built up in layers. Second – and more importantly – you gradually learn how to build your **own** documents. The Wizard is, in fact, an excellent and almost subliminal teacher.

The help does not stop there. You can choose to work with Cue Cards during your work period with the program. These are help screens that pop up on the screen to offer you tips or to make suggestions about how you might layout the next part of your document. Once you become familiar with Publisher, these become annoying. No problem. You simply turn this feature off. Other help comes in the form of 'tips' that are attached to many help screens and offers of demonstrations'. If you make a mistake, the program asks you if you would like to be 'shown' how to do a certain operation.

All of this works **on top** of an extremely powerful desktop publishing program. Publisher is a fully featured program that allows you to manipulate text to degrees unheard off a few years ago. It enables you to create formal and less formal creations that will enhance the quality of the documents that you produce on your PC. You can import text from other programs (such as Word for Windows and you can insert pictures, tables and all of the other objects that go to make up designed documents. You can layout books and reports, newsletters and advertisements, design conference posters and flyers and develop your own corporate logos and stationery.

Page Plus

Like Publisher, described above, **Page Plus** is another desktop publishing program. It is more powerful than Publisher but, arguably, not quite so easy to use.

Page Plus runs under Windows and calls for a computer with at least a 386 processor, 3 mb of memory and 5 mb of free hard-disk space. It installs, easily from five high-density disks and can be set up to run in three different modes – at three different levels of complexity. This is a particularly good system. As you get used to using the program, so you can take on a little more of it and so some of the 'help' offered is reduced. Page Plus runs close to the wire on the help issue. It has various means of offering help and some of these can be turned off. It is possible to feel 'overhelped' with all of the help devices turned on.

The program does all that you expect from a desktop publisher. You can produce pages of text in the program's integrated word processor and then layout that text on single pages. You can also import clip art (small illustrations) and text and pictures in other formats. You can also change the default black and white settings for multicolour if you have a colour printer (and these are becoming much cheaper to buy). Colour is particularly useful in single-page flyers and for preparing overhead projection acetates.

Page Plus does not use all of the 'Windows conventions' that have grown up around programs that work under Windows and this can sometimes be frustrating. Sometimes, rather than working intuitively, you have to stop and think about how to achieve something on the screen. Not that all this is difficult: merely that there are still details that can be improved. Overall, this is an extremely well thought out product and one that helps you to produce professional looking copy very easily. As always with desktop publishing programs, the secret – if there is one – is to keep things **simple**. Faced with an array of fonts in different sizes and the ability to manipulate text and pictures in all sorts of ways, there is a temptation to get carried away. All of the books on graphic design stress the simplicity rule. Stick to it and Page Plus will help you to write your brochures and catalogues as well as conference programs and teaching aids.

Project

Developing and planning long- and short-term projects used to involve graph paper and complicated wall charts. Now you can get your projects organized, much more efficiently, with a computer program. **Microsoft Project** is what it says: a program for organizing all elements of any type of project. Health care professionals are likely to find it particularly useful for organizing research projects, organizational change, long-term management development, trials, conferences and curriculum plans. There are three phases to project management. First, you create the project. This is, traditionally, the 'brainstorming' phase. Project allows you to play around with possibilities and then to structure a framework for organizing the project. Second, you **manage** the project. Project allows you to keep track of all the elements of your project, to predict problems, to reallocate time and make all sorts of fine adjustments. Third, you produce reports of the project. Again, Project helps here by creating informative and attractive reports quickly and easily.

The project management techniques that Project offer are comprehensive. You can use the Critical Path Method of scheduling – an approach already in use by many managers. Or you can use the Program Evaluation Review Technique (PERT) – another method that has often been used in the health care professions to organize and manage the use of time. Finally, you can use Gantt Charts – perhaps the most familiar way of illustrating time-spans in a project.

Initially, you can enter 'events' in your project into a spreadsheet-type screen. Then you can reorder events, retime them, reschedule them and manipulate those events to a considerable degree. Various views of your data allow you different perspectives on your project. The business of working with Project takes you far beyond a mere paper exercise. The program can help you develop and think through both large and small projects. Fund-holders will appreciate being able to time and cost sections of projects and know that they can always run projects of the 'what-if?' sort.

This is not a program to load up and work with immediately. You have to invest a little effort in getting to know it. Fortunately, as with many new Microsoft programs, a good deal of help is at hand. First, you get a run-through of the main points of the program when you first start it up. Then, you can have the program 'talk you through' the various elements of project design and scheduling. Finally, you can call up context-sensitive help at any time. Also, the reference manual is excellent and informative. Microsoft produce **readable** manuals. These are not simply alphabetical lists of what programs do. Instead, they are laid out in easy to follow and easy to digest chapters.

Project is highly compatible with other Windows programs and particularly with other Microsoft programs. If you already use Word for Windows or Excel, you will soon get used to Project. It uses the Common User Interface that runs throughout the Microsoft range of programs and honours all of the 'Windows conventions'.

SPREADSHEETS

A spreadsheet program allows you to develop a huge 'rows and columns' chart on your computer. It does more than this: it also allows you to undertake a whole range of calculations on each or on a selection of the rows and columns. In some ways it is like a computerized and automated accounts book. On the other hand, it can also do far more than just compute rows and columns. It can be used for at least the following functions too:

- for storing addresses;
- for compiling bibliographies and reference lists;
- for drawing 'word illustrations' in column format;
- for computing frequency counts;
- for working out means and modes.

Figure 3.1 is an example of what a spreadsheet looks like when it has data in it.

	A	B	C	D
1	Response to Question Six (Health care professionals should receive more training in the field of child abuse)			
2		Social workers	Doctors	Nurses
3	Agree	23	37	56
4	Disagree	10	8	10
5	Don't know	0	3	5

Figure 3.1

Examples of spreadsheet programs that are available commercially include the following:

- Excel for Windows
- Lotus 123
- PC Planner
- Quattro
- Supercalc

GRAPHICS

Graphics packages allow you to illustrate and generally 'dress up' your work. A top commercial package will help you to do the following:

- generate graphs, histograms and pie charts;
- use 'clip art' to illustrate news letters and projects;
- make slide presentations;
- generate charts for use as overhead projections in teaching;
- draw organization charts.

A good graphics program can help to make your work look more professional and can help you to communicate your thoughts through iconic representation. A basic rule applies here, though: keep it simple. Graphics programs can generate very complicated illustrations and diagrams. It is easy to get carried away with what they can do. Generally communication is much clearer if you stick to simple charts and representations.

Examples of graphics programs that are available commercially include the following:

- Animator
- Applause
- Arts and Letters
- Corel Draw
- Freelance Graphics
- Harvard Graphics

A WRITER'S SOFTWARE STARTER KIT

So what **must** you have in the way of software? This chapter has offered descriptions of quite a few programs: it is sometimes difficult to know what sorts of programs are absolutely essential. Here is a shortlist of programs recommended for anyone who wants to set their computer up for writing.

A word processor

Clearly essential. You are not going to write very much with your computer if you do not have one of these. As we have seen, there is a considerable range to choose from. If you are new to computing, one of the 'smaller' ones will be quite adequate and you may even find that the program **Write** – which is supplied with Windows – is sufficient. It can certainly enable you to carry out all the basic functions of producing, editing and printing out documents.

A utilities program

Everyone has hard-disk problems at some point in their computing career. Such problems often seem to arise just when you do not need them. When they do happen, you need a utilities program to get you out of trouble. Such programs can help you to find files, restore the integrity of your hard disk, compress files and so on. Examples of utilities programs include Norton Utilities (described in this chapter) and PC Tools.

A simple database program

You will want to store bibliographical references as you write. As we have seen, you can use a variety of programs for this purpose. Simplicity is probably the keyword here. What you do not want to do is to have to learn a complicated program simply in order to file away your references. Various programs have been described in this chapter and a number of dedicated bibliographical programs are available as shareware.

A graphics package

This is not essential but is very useful if you need to make diagrams and tables to go with your writing.

An uninstall program

Most writers produce large numbers of text files. Many word-processing programs make backup files as the user works with the program. With hard-disk space at a premium for most users, the uninstall program is becoming an essential one for writers. The program **Clean Sweep** is described in this chapter but plenty of others are also available.

COPYRIGHT

Remember that all software is copyright. You cannot simply borrow someone else's disks and then copy them onto your machine. If you are going to use a program you must buy it. Mostly, the copyright agreement on software is rather like the copyright attached to books. Only one person at a time can read a book and you must not photocopy the book. The same goes for software. Only one person at a time should be able to use a particular program.

SHAREWARE

Shareware has a unique marketing strategy. A shareware program is distributed free of charge (although a charge is usually made for the disks and the handling). The idea is that you first try the program and then, if you like it, you send away a registration fee to use the program. In the first instance, you usually have between 30 and 90 days to try out the program before you register it. Further, during this time, you are encouraged to make copies of the program for your colleagues and friends. Then, the same principles apply: they are allowed to try out the program and then send off to become registered users if they find it useful.

The advantages of the shareware approach are many for the home PC user. First, she gets a chance to try the program before making a financial commitment to it. Second, the registration fees for shareware are considerably cheaper than buying copies of most commercial programs. Also, the quality of shareware programs is improving all the time and some of the best is easily the equal of commercial software. Finally, shareware offers you the easy approach to learning more about computer programs and to explore a variety of methods of working with data that you may not have been able to if you had to rely on buying commercial packages. The names and addresses of shareware distributors are available in any of the monthly computer magazines. Such magazine offers include one or two shareware programs on a 'free' disk attached to the front cover.

Shareware is not free. The idea, as we noted above, is to try out the program, decide if you like it and then pay for it. If you decide not to use the program then you simply give the disks to another person or format the disks for use with other files. The only free programs are those available in the Public Domain. These public domain programs are often distributed by the same people that handle shareware although it is often not made clear in their catalogues what is shareware and what is public domain. The following is a short selection of examples of shareware programs that may be of particular interest to the writer. This is necessarily a limited selection: there are thousands of programs to choose from.

Outline

This is, as the name suggests, an outlining program. It allows you to 'brainstorm' ideas, straight onto the computer and then to sort them under headings and sub headings. I have used this program and found the idea of it very good. In practice, though, I found that it was just as easy brainstorming with a word processor. Outline is a very professional and very detailed program that, if you like it, is worth learning.

Galaxy Lite

This is a shareware word processor. It is very easy to use and has many of the functions of expensive commercial packages. It's one big failing is that it does not have a word counter – an indispensable aid to a writer. On the other hand, the program runs in a very small amount of memory and loads very quickly. I have used this program on my laptop computer.

Sharespell

This is a stand-alone spell-checker containing more than 112 000 words. It is ideal for use with Galaxy Lite and enables you to have an almost complete word-processing system.

Cliché Finder

This finds your clichés for you. I have listed some clichés to avoid as an appendix to this book. This program weeds out some of the worst ones from your writing. You can also enter your own phrases into the program and it will seek them out in the text that you run through it.

Idea Tree

This is a unique and powerful thinking tool. It allows you to break down concepts into component parts and then to reassemble the various component in different formats. Similar, in a way, to the Outline but a program that works in a very different way.

Jorj Dictionary

An on-board computer dictionary that can operate as a stand-alone program or as a Terminate and Stay Resident one. A Terminate and Stay Resident program loads into the memory of your computer and you can then pop it up over the program that you are working in. For example, you may be writing in your word-processing program and want to check the meaning of a word. You push a couple of buttons and you are in the dictionary. You push a couple more and you are back in your word processor. This dictionary has about 58 000 words.

Express Graph

A shareware graphics program that is not quite as powerful as many of its commercial counterparts. This one can draw graphs, bar charts and exploded pie charts. Graphs from this program can be printed out to any EPSON-compatible printer (which includes quite a few).

Flashback

All through this chapter, I have pointed up the importance of backing up the data on your hard disk. This simple to use program is one that allows you to do this without having to work through the sometimes complicated file copying programs that come with your operating system.

Flexibak

This is another flexible, efficient and easy to use hard-disk backup system. All of these sorts of programs save you time and frustration and you are recommended to get one.

Maxiread

This is one of a number of programs that checks your work for style. As usual, this program tends to compare your work with American standards of English so you have to be a little careful if you are writing in 'English English'.

Multiword

This is an electronic thesaurus. If your current word processor does not have a thesaurus facility, this one is excellent.

New York Word

This is a word-processing program that can rival many of the larger commercial packages. It contains many of the features of those programs and is worth considering if you want an inexpensive word processor.

PC-Type

This is another word-processing program from the Brown Bag company and it is both simple to use and yet has most of the essential elements that a word processor should have. With PC-Type you can work with up to ten documents at once.

RGB Techwriter

This is the word processor for those who do a lot of technical writing. It is specially designed to make technical typing involving the input of complex symbolic expressions fast, easy and accurate.

Project Management

This is a projects organizer and helps you to keep track of a timetable of events. It may be useful for anyone conducting research and for those who are responsible for keeping track of other people's work.

This is a sample of some of the programs that you may find useful in the shareware domain. Remember, though, that the programs are not free. As has been suggested, you pay, initially, for the cost of the disk and for the copying.

After that, you have about 30–90 days to evaluate the program before sending off your registration fee. All this is down to trust. You **can** carry on using the program but you are morally obliged to send off your registration fee. Apparently, not so many people do in the UK as do in the USA. For this reason, some American shareware companies have stopped trading in the UK.

CD-ROMS

CD-ROMs (Compact Disc: Read Only Memory) are compact discs that contain up to about 600 mb of information. As the name suggests, most of them can only be 'read' by the computer – they cannot be written to. Increasingly, this situation is changing and machines are being produced that write to as well as read CDs. While, at the time of writing, many CD-ROMs contain games, educational material for children, some are available that are useful to the writer. Many commercial programs such as word processors and graphics packages now come on CD-ROM. This saves having to load a a program onto your hard disk from a large number of floppy disks. Instead, you insert the CD-ROM and instruct your computer to load the new program onto your computer's hard disk. You can then go away and let the computer do the rest.

Not all new computers come complete with a CD player but many now do. Lots of people feel that they are worth the investment and are worth buying as an 'add on'. To get the best out of CD-ROMS (and, in some cases, to make them work at all) you need a certain specification of computer. The Multimedia PC Marketing Council has laid down the following two standards as the minimum requirements for working with CD-ROMs and other multimedia. They are referred to as Level 1 and Level 2.

Level 1: the entry-level standard

- **processor**: 386SX CPU with 2 mb RAM, 30 mb hard disk, serial, parallel, MIDI i/o and joystick ports, mouse;
- **display**: VGA display adaptor and monitor at 640 × 480 resolution; technically, 16 colours is the minimum requirement but 256 is recommended and is used by most MPC programs;
- **sound system**: 8-bit wave audio at 22 kHz using no more than 19% of the CPU capacity; MIDI (music synthesizer) with the ability to play back multi-voice, multi-timbral sounds, 6 melody notes and 2 percussive notes simultaneously; ability to mix CD audio, synthesizer and wave sounds into one stereo line out;
- **CD-ROM drive**: capable of transferring data at a sustained rate of 150 kb per second using not more than 40% of CPU capacity; average seek time better than 1 second; CD digital audio outpus with volume control;
- **software**: Windows 3.0 with the multimedia extensions or later (i.e. Windows 3.1 or 3.11). MSCDEX version 2.2 or greater.

Level 2: the higher level

As level 1, above, plus the following hardware enhnacements:

- **processor**: 486SX/25 mHz CPU, 4 mb RAM (8 mb recommended) 160 mb hard drive;
- **display**: VGA-compatible adapter with 640 × 480 pixel resolution in 65 536 colours;
- **sound system**: 16-bit wave audio at 44.1 kHz sampling rate in mono and stereo; no more than 10% of CPU time should be needed to play 22.05 kHz sounds; no more than 15% of CPU time should be needed to play 44.1 kHz audio;
- **CD-ROM drive**: CD-ROM drive with a sustained data rate of 300 kb per second using no more than 50% of CPU time; the average seek time must be 400 milliseconds of less; the drive must be multisession and XA ready.

If you are planning to add a CD-ROM to your computer, you are advised to meet the later specification, as a minimum, if at all possible. You can also use the specifications for checking the products that you consider or as information for the person who fits your CD-ROM equipment.

Here are some CD-ROM programs that will be of value to the writer.

Encarta

This is a fully interactive, 28-volume encyclopaedia with over 17 000 multimedia elements, including text, pictures, animations and sounds. It includes a full text searching facilitity and the means of cross-referencing and cross-searching.

Grolier Multimedia Encyclopaedia

This is another impressive encyclopaedia on disk. It contains over six hours of mutlimedia presentations which include 8000 pictures, a graphical 'timeline', fact boxes, fully interactive essays, pictures and sounds.

Oxford Reference Shelf on CD-ROM

This has been described as a set of programs elsewhere in this book. The whole suite of programs is also available as a single CD-ROM. The disc contains *The Pocket Oxford Dictionary*, *The Oxford Dictionary for Writers and Editors*, *The Oxford Guide to English Usage*, *The Oxford Mini-Dictionary of Quotations*, a *Compact Encylopaedia*, a *Concise Dictionary of Business*, a *Concise Dictionary of Law*, *The Oxford Dictionary of Abbreviations*, a *World Gazetteer*, *The Oxford French Mini-Dictionary*, *The Oxford German Mini-Dictionary*, *The Oxford Spanish Mini-Dictionary*, *The Oxford Italian Mini-Dictionary*, a *Concise Dictionary of Science*, *The Oxford Dictionary for Scientific Writers and*

Editors and *The Oxford Dictionary of Computing*. All in all, a comprehensive library of reference books in a very compact format.

Concise Oxford Dictionary

This is another program that is also available as a set of floppy disks. This CD-ROM contains the entire **Concise Oxford Dictionary** on disc and has a fast and easy-to-use searching facility.

Justis Environmental Health CD-ROM

This disc offers synopses of UK and EC legislation, regulations and guidelines on environmental control and health and safety issues. The disc is updated every six months to reflect changes in legislation.

Bookfind-CD World Edition

This contains a listing of books currently available with all relevant information such as author, date of publication, title, ISBN number and publisher, together with a description of the contents of each publication. This is available with monthly updates and is not particularly cheap but will be an ideal resource for institutions and colleges. There is also a Medical and Health Care edition available.

The Guardian, *The Times*, the *Telegraph*, the *International Herald Tribune*

All of these papers are available as 'years' and often as 'decades' on CD-ROM.

Databases are dealt with in Chapter 5. All writers need them and they deserve a chapter to themselves. But now it's time to look at the business itself – of writing with a computer.

Writing with a computer | 4

There is no such thing as a moral or an immoral book. Books are well written, or badly written.

Oscar Wilde

The point is to write. Computers may seem to take away some of the romance and the mystery of writing but they can help you no end. The previous chapter offered reasons for using a computer in writing and described some of the software that is available for personal computers. In this chapter, we identify some of the issues related to writing with the use of a computer. It is assumed that you have chosen the word processor of your choice and that you have got used to the fundamentals of it. You have, perhaps, passed the stage that the writer Primo Levi describes as he writes of beginning to use a computer and word processor:

> If I now analyse my initial anxiety, I realize that it was in great part illogical: it contained an old fear of those who write, the fear that the unique, inestimable text worked at so hard, which will give you eternal fame, might be stolen or end up in a manhole. Here you write, the words appear neatly on the screen, well aligned, but they are shadows: they are immaterial, deprived of the reassuring support of the paper. The written word speaks out: the screen does not; when you are satisfied with the text 'you put it on disk', where it becomes invisible. Is it still there, absconding in some little corner of the memory disk, or did you destroy it with some mistaken move? (Levi, 1989)

HOUSEKEEPING

The word, in this context, is used to denote those activities that are concerned with the management of computer files and the hard disk. It is tempting, when you first get a computer with a hard disk, to simply pile all of your software onto it in no particular order. This is fatal. If you do this, you will be unable to find which files belong to which programs. Instead, you make use of the hierarchical faculty of the operating system that you are using: DOS or Windows.

The first process is to decide what directories you need. It is usual to keep nothing in the 'root' directory (on the hard disk, this is usually drive c:) other than the autoexec.bat, config.sys files and the bare necessities of the operating system itself. With those in the root, you open subdirectories. It is useful to see these in terms of a pyramid. If the root is the tip of the pyramid, then the next layer of subdirectories contain your program directories. In the next layer, as subdirectories of the program directories, you have your data directories. Figure 4.1 illustrates this set of relationships.

The root (c:\) Contains only files to start up computer			
c:\ word Directory containing your wordprocessing files		c:\datab Directory containing your database files	
c:\word\data 1 Data files	c:\word\data 2 Data files	c:\datab\data 1 Data files	c:\datab\data 2 Data files

Figure 4.1

Essentially, you keep your word-processing program files in one subdirectory and your database program files in another. As two branches of your word-processing subdirectory, you have two (or more) subdirectories in which you keep your data. The same system is true for database directories. You open a new subdirectory for every program you keep on your hard disk and you open further subdirectories for the data files that you create with those programs. If you are uncertain about how to do this, consult the handbook that comes with your operating system or with your programs. Many programs run an installation routine. When you put the first floppy disk in the drive, the program asks you if you would like a new subdirectory opened for the program files to go into. The installation program then creates a new subdirectory on your hard disk and unpacks all the new program files into it.

Some people prefer to keep subdirectories to a minimum. Instead of subdirectories within the program directories, they keep such directories completely-separate. For example, they will have a system which branches as shown in Figure 4.2

Root directory (c:\)		
C:\word Wordprocessing files	C:\datab Database files	C:\data Data files

Figure 4.2

This system is often simpler. It is also quicker to operate. As a general rule, the fewer 'levels' of directories that you have, the quicker your computer will work. As in most things, the keywords are simplicity and structure.

Housekeeping also refers to making sure that you know what is on your hard disk. Make frequent checks to see what files you have made and which ones you **have** to keep on your hard disk. Do not keep files on the hard disk that you never use. Also, clear off any files that are cluttering up your data directories. It is easy, especially when you are new to computing, to open up various 'trial' files: ones that you experiment with. Make sure that they are wiped off periodically.

Most of all, housekeeping refers to the process of backing up your hard disk. Put simply, this means that everything that is on your hard disk should also be on floppies. All of your program files will already be on floppies for that is the medium on which you brought them. Any data files that you make will need backing up as you create them. It is a good idea to get into the habit of backing up at the end of each working session on the computer. Programs are available that will back up any new files that have been made, automatically. All you have to do is to invoke the program, put a new floppy disk in the appropriate drive and press a couple of buttons. The program will then do what is called an 'incremental' backup. The only files that are backed up are new ones or ones that have be written to since the last backup. Alternatively, you can use one of the copying programs that come within DOS or Windows. Also, many discrete programs have backup facilities. WordPerfect, for example, allows you to back up files through its 'file manager' feature. All you have to do is to highlight any new or modified files and ask for copies to be made to floppy disk.

Backing up the hard disk is essential. All hard disks fail at some time. You are only a limited amount of time away from the hard disk failing completely. If it does this, you stand to loose all of the files that are on it. If you backup your work, you can always find the files and the work that you need. That work is always ready on floppy disks, even when you cannot use the hard disk.

If you make lots of changes to files, or delete files and make new ones, after a while, the hard disk becomes fragmented. Files are scattered on different parts of the disk. After about 6 months, it is useful to run a program that 'optimizes' the hard disk and pushes all the files together on the disk, closing up the small gaps that exist between them. No harm occurs to the files but your hard disk runs more quickly and efficiently. The brute force way of dealing with this problem is to backup the whole of the hard disk, to reformat it and then to load all the backed up files back onto the hard disk. In this way, all the files line up, one next to the other and all the gaps are closed up. Fragmentation is not a major problem and many people live for years without giving it a thought. If you want your system to run as quickly and as efficiently as it can, though, it is worth thinking about how you will cope when the hard disk does get fragmented. Tell-tale signs are slow reading of the hard disk accompanied by the hard disk spinning a considerable amount every time a file is read to or from it. As mentioned on pp. 48 and 49, Norton Utilities and PC Tools both have a 'speed disk' feature which repairs disk fragmentation.

SETTING UP YOUR WORD PROCESSOR

Most of the larger word processors can be configured to work the way that you want them to. They all have 'default' settings: standard settings that allow you to work with the program straight away. On the other hand, you can change many of these defaults in order to have the word processor work the way **you** want it. Examples of defaults that you can reset and have running with new definitions include the following:

- **Colours**   The rule, as ever, is simplicity. Do not overwhelm yourself with too many colour combinations. Use the same colour to indicate various degrees of 'large' fonts. Don't allocate a different colour to each function or you will quickly forget what your colour scheme means. Also, have a change of background colour, occasionally.
- **Right and left margins**   You can have wide settings for these when you are working at the screen and then change them for printing out. The wide margins when you are working will allow your eyes to scan a single line at a time and thus save you constantly turning your head back and forward. Also, some word-processing programs cause the writing to go off the edge of the screen if you use only 1 in margins. Reset them so that you can see all of what you have written.
- **Top and bottom margins**   For work that you submit for publication, allow fairly generous margins all round. I have mine set to 1.5 in for top, bottom and sides.
- **Tab settings**   If you want to get things exactly right, the correct setting for 'indents' at the beginning of paragraphs is two or three 'ems'. An em is the width of a single character. It is possible on some of the larger word processors to set the first tab setting to ensure that all of your indents are two or three ems.
- **Backup settings**   Modern word processors automatically backup the file that you are working on to the hard disk, at pre-set intervals. You can set the time limit for this. You must **still** make regular backups of your hard disk files to floppies.
- **Font sizes**   Most word processors allow you to work in different sized letters and numbers. With some, you may see the difference on the screen.
- **Underlining style**   Words and spaces or just words. It is usual to underline both words and spaces. If you are printing out on a laser printer, you may prefer to use italics rather than underlining in your work. In a manuscript, underlining is used to represent passages that will be printed as italics in the final publication. I have changed my 'underlining' command on my word processor to produce italics, automatically. This stops me having to think whether or not I want underlining or italics. Nothing is for ever: the underlining function can soon be returned to normal if this should be important at a later date.
- **Paper and page size**   There is only one size paper for writing: A4. Do not

use smaller or larger sizes. Also, buy fairly good paper of about 80 gms in weight. For posting work to publishers, do not use heavier paper than this otherwise your bill for stamps will be rather large. Use plain paper and not 'laid'. Laid paper has feint lines running through it in the style of a watermark.

- **Page numbering**
- **Headers and footers** (and the contents of these)   Use these sparingly. Although printed books and magazines have running headers and footers it is not a good idea to use them in manuscripts that you send to editors. They only have to cross them through when they are editing your work. On the other hand, with book manuscripts, it is good practice to have a simple header that contains your name and the title of the book. This is useful if the editor or anyone else leaves half of your manuscript in the office and half at home. Without any sort of identification, it may be difficult to marry the two piles of paper together.
- **Keyboard layout**   Some word processors allow you to modify your keyboard considerably.
- **Justification**   You may prefer to have both margins flush or to have the words at the right margin 'ragged'. Generally speaking, laser printed pages look better with justification turned on, while dot matrix printed pages looked better with it turned off ('ragged right').
- **Column and/or table settings**
- **Line spacing**   If you are submitting work for publication, always double space it.
- **Buttons**   Many Windows word-processing packages allow you to set up 'buttons' at the top of the screen which, when 'pressed' with the mouse, trigger certain functions.

There are many more types of default settings that you can reset.

Many word processors allow you to write 'macros'. Consider, for a moment, a function of your word processor that requires you to work through lots of keystrokes in order to invoke the function. A macro is a 'shorthand' that allows you to assign all of those keystrokes to just two keystrokes. For example, on the keyboard that I am working on at present, if I press ALT and S, the word processor will run the spell-checker. These keypresses are not standard: first I had to write the macros that make them function in that way. It is possible to build up a considerable collection of such macros that allow you to invoke functions quickly and easily. It is worth taking a little time to learn the macro language that accompanies your word processor.

With some word processors it is also possible to reassign keys to function according to your own preference. None of this is irreversible. Don't get nervous about what could happen if you make mistakes. It is always possible to reinstate the normal function of the keys that you change.

WORKING WITH A WORD PROCESSOR

There are a number of tips that can make writing easier with a word processor. These are itemized, below. Try to standardize the way that you work so that your output is consistent. If you decide, for example, to use 2 in margins when you write essays, **always** use 2 in margins. Consider resetting the margin defaults to 2 in, so that every piece of writing you produce has 2 in margins. This sort of standardization is important. Here are the tips for working with your word processor:

- Although your final output will usually be in double-spaced lines, use single-spaced lines to work with on your screen. Double line spacing on the monitor means that you effectively halve the amount of text you can see on the screen at any one time.
- If you can, experiment with the speed of your cursor. If necessary, reset the speed according to the work that you are doing. If, for example, you are scrolling through a long document, set the cursor speed to high. If you are doing word by word or line by line editing, slow the cursor down. Not all word processors allow you to change the speed of the cursor.
- Work with small documents. You do not need to keep the whole of a piece of work in one file. Large documents take time to work through. It may be better to split a large document into two separate files.
- When working on large documents, set the margin settings wide. This will mean that there are fewer words on each line on the screen. This will allow you to scan lines of text more easily. You can change the margin size back to normal when you have finished editing.
- Be consistent. Pay particular attention to your use of underlining, bolding and italics. Don't mix the three. Settle for one type of emphasis and stick to it.
- Be consistent in your line spacing between ends of sections and new subheadings. As a rule, leave two lines between the end of a section and a new subheading. Then leave one line between the subheading and the text.
- Be careful about indenting paragraphs. Do not indent the first paragraph of a piece of work, nor subsequent first paragraphs under subheadings. After that, indent every paragraph. For an immediate example of both line spacing and indentation, look at the use of both in this book. This book is laid out according to the standard rules governing page layout.
- Be consistent with your use of full stops and commas. It is not always necessary to use commas in a 'bullet' list (such as this one). If you do use them, use them consistently.
- Avoid mixing up different fonts on a page. It is not good practice to use all the different sizes of numbers and figures that your word processor will allow. Keep to one or two sizes. As a rule, 12 pt is a good size font to use for everyday writing. Also, Times/Roman is a clear and clean font if you have a laser printer. Fashions in typefaces come and go. At the moment, sans serif fonts (those without 'tails' on the letters) tend to be out of fashion. Times/Roman seems to be something of a standard font.

- Don't overuse graphics. If your word processor can use 'clip art' or pre-drawn pieces of drawing and illustration, use it very sparingly, if at all.
- If you can work in more than one document at a time and have a coloured screen, change the background colours in the second and third document screens. In this way, you are less likely to be muddled up about which document you are working on.
- Save your work regularly. That means that you have to stop typing and consciously save your work to the hard disk. Again, later on, copy your new file to a floppy so that you always have a backed up version of it.
- Name your files with recognizable names. When naming chapter files, for a book like this, I try to use both a number (which indicates the chapter number) and a short name (which indicates what the chapter is about). The file name for this chapter is: 4WRITECO – shorthand for 'Chapter Four: Writing with Computers'. Develop your own codes but don't stick to using only numbers. You will never remember what the numbers stand for. Some word processors allow you to use 'long names'. WordPerfect, for example, allows you to use a name of up to 32 characters. Using WordPerfect, it would be quite possible to name this file: 'Chapter Four: Writing: Computers'.
- Use 'odd' names for temporary files that you use for blocks of text or for ideas. I tend to use the file names 'Dog' and 'Cat' for these sorts of files. When I am 'housekeeping' I know that these are files that I can delete.
- If you are referring to names of authors and dates, while writing essays or articles, and cannot remember those names and dates as you write, use a consistent symbol to note the place where they should go. I use three asterisks (***). Then, using the 'search' facility, you can go straight to those symbols after you have finished writing and fill in the blanks. Thus, when I am writing, a section of the text may look like this:

> Student-centred learning owes much to the work of Carl Rogers (***). The idea that adult learners might want to be responsible for their learning was also discussed by Malcolm Knowles (***) and Postman and Weingartner (***).

Then, I simply search for the ***s and insert the correct dates.

- Write quickly and edit later. If you find that your spelling suffers a little, don't worry too much, you can always correct this with the spell-checker. If this seems a sloppy approach, remember: the word processor is there to save you time – use it. If you find it helps, use a shorthand for words that you find difficult to spell. For instance, you might use 'exp' for the term 'experiential', if you found that word tricky to spell. When you have finished writing, the spell-checker will soon flag this 'non-word' up and you will be offered the correct spelling for it. It is quite possible to become much faster at writing through developing a personal shorthand of this sort.
- A variant of the above is to use letters for complicated names. For example,

if you are writing an essay about Dostoevsky but find the name difficult to spell and remember, simply type the letters DY. Then use the search and replace command to replace those letters with the full name, throughout your manuscript.

- Try to learn most of the function of your word processor and learn all the shortcuts. I once found a colleague working through a file on the screen, inserting 'hard returns' between each line of text to ensure that the manuscript printed out in double spacing. He did not realize that he could set the word processor to print in double spacing.
- If your word processor has a thesaurus, use it regularly to give you ideas for different words. This can not only teach you words but it can freshen your writing.
- Avoid footnotes and endnotes in documents, even if your word processor can handle them automatically. If you have anything that you want to put as a footnote, incorporate it into the main body of the text. Otherwise, leave it out altogether. Footnotes are always distracting.[1] An exception to this rule is discussed in Chapter 8.
- If you can, run off a draft 'hard' copy of your work before you submit it. It is often easier to spot typographical errors on the printed page than it is on the computer screen.
- Don't work for long periods at the computer. If you **have** to, work on different documents. It is a great strain to both eyes and posture if you work for hours on one document. Look away from the screen when the computer is busy working at a particular function. Get used to getting up and walking around the room at regular intervals. Take long coffee or tea breaks.

LEARNING TO TYPE

This is a contentious point but if you are going to be serious about writing, it may be a good idea to learn to type. It seems odd to have a very fast and powerful computer coupled to a state-of-the-art word-processing program only to use it to 'hunt and peck' for the keys. There are numerous typing courses available in colleges and as evening classes. There are also some excellent do-it-yourself teaching packages available for use on the computer. One of the best is the interestingly named *Mavis Beacon Teaches Typing*. Being able to touch type and to use all of your fingers really does speed up the way you use a computer for writing. It also frees you up to think, not about the keyboard, but about the ideas that you have.

1. There! Even this one is distracting, even though it has nothing in it. Few people can resist reading what is in a footnote.

Keeping databases

'You must begin by making notes. You may have to make notes for years ... When you think of something, when you recall something, put it where it belongs,' he said. 'Put it down when you think of it. You may never recapture it quite as vividly the second time.'

F. Scott Fitzgerald

All writers need to keep notes. Some need to keep very specific notes: notes of the books and articles they have written. This chapter is all about how to store information that you need in formats that will enable you to find it again. I admit to working with huge piles of papers. The desk I am sitting at is covered with papers. On the other hand, if I want to find out what books I have read on counselling since 1985, I only have to press a couple of buttons on the computer to find out. The important thing is to organize some of your chaos – even if you don't organize all of it. When preparing to write this chapter I was struck by the number of books on writing that suggest that you carefully organize **all** of your information by using elaborate filing systems and methods of cross reference. A couple of those books' writers were frank enough to admit that 'of course, **I** don't work that way myself ... I am much less organized.' Yet this struck me as a bit dishonest. Find a system that suits you and stick to it. Don't get caught up in the interesting but distracting business of building an elaborate database that **should** allow you to find whatever you want but which takes up so much time in maintenance that it is hardly worth the bother. As before, the keywords are simplicity and structure.

WHAT IS A DATABASE?

Simply, a database is an organized collection of information. The word tends to be associated with computer programs that file away information but that definition limits its use. It is also used to mean **a** system that allows you to store and retrieve information.

USES OF DATABASES

For the writer, the obvious use of a database is for the storing of bibliographical references. Over the years, I have developed a store of about 1000 such references. Originally, I used a system of cards. Now I use what is called a 'free-form database' program. I will explain the use of both of these methods and others. Also, a writer and researcher can use databases for the following:

- storing and retrieving interview data;
- storing and retrieving numerical data;
- keeping odd bits of information that are not easily classified;
- storing ideas for papers, articles, research projects and books;
- storing quotable quotes;
- analysing qualitative data;
- storing and retrieving names and addresses;
- keeping track of a project;
- collecting and executing 'to do' lists.

Databases also have lots of other uses and can be used by teachers and practitioners to store details of lectures, case notes and other information that needs to be referred to frequently. Remember, though, if you are going to store personal information about people, you will need to clarify your position regarding the Data Protection Act. You cannot simply store personal information about other people in a computer file. You must first be sure that you are not contravening the Act.

STORING BIBLIOGRAPHIC REFERENCES

The most simple way of keeping a reference database is by writing the details of the reference on an index card and storing it in a plastic box. Various sorts of cards and various sorts of boxes are available in any branch of W. H. Smith's or any stationers. In my experience, most people like buying stationery so this, initial, part of the process is usually a pleasant one. It is usually preferable to go for the larger 8 × 5 in cards. These allow you more space for notes.

The card system works like this. You lay out the card as in Figure 5.1. Then you file the card, alphabetically, using index dividers that you can buy with your box. Later on, when you want to find all your references by a particular author, you simply look up the author's name and find all the references that you need.

Another filing method is to keep duplicate cards and use a keyword system. Thus, on the relevant cards, you write COUNSELLING or SOCIAL POLICY and file these together. As long as you know your keywords (and you keep a note of these on a separate card at the front of your box) you can collect together a range of references on a particular topic, quickly and easily. Life gets more complicated. What happens with a book like Carl Rogers's *On Becoming a Person*? Do you file it under COUNSELLING or PSYCHOTHERAPY or, perhaps PSYCHOLOGY? This is where it soon becomes worth considering using a computerized system. Don't rush, too quickly, to use one, though. I have heard of people setting up reference databases with such heavyweight programs such as Dbase or Paradox. While it is entirely possible to do this, there may be simpler ways of working.

First of all, though, the illustration of how to complete a reference card. The elements of the card are always the same:

- the name of the surname of the author and her initials;
- the year of publication;
- the title of the book or paper;
- the publisher or name of the journal;
- the place of publication or the edition and page numbers of the journal;
- keywords;
- comments.

Figure 5.1 offers two examples: the reference card for a book and the reference card for a journal article. You are free, of course, to modify this format to suit yourself. Once you have settled on a format, stick to it.

Using this card format, it is also possible to write direct quotations from the publications straight onto the card for quotation in your essay or article. Two things are important here. First, make sure that you write down the quote exactly as it appears in the book or paper. Make no attempt to tidy up the grammar or spelling. You must leave quotations as they are. Second, make sure you write down the page number. When you use direct quotations in essays and research reports (and you should use them sparingly) you must always state the page number. Thus, a reference to a direct quotation from the first reference in the illustration above might look like this:

Used skilfully, gestalt therapy is an arresting, often oblique form of dialogue which involves a wide range of techniques. (Smith, 1995: 53)

You may not like the grammar nor the language but you must leave the quotation exactly as the author wrote it. Also, avoid using the word *sic* to denote that this is a direct quotation and that you are aware of its shortcomings.

As your reference database grows, it will outgrow the plastic container you spent so much time choosing in W. H. Smith's. You then have a number of choices:

- buy another plastic container and begin to fill that up;
- buy a filing drawer: this will take you years to fill up;
- consider computerizing your system.

```
Smith, P.
1995
Learning Interactive Skills: a Reflective Guide
for Health Care Professionals, 3rd edition,
Butterworth-Heinemann, Oxford.

Keywords: self-awareness, experiential learning,
exercises

Comments: Source of activities for learning a
range of interpersonal and communication skills.
Aimed at nurses but also relevant to other health
professionals.
```

Figure 5.1a Reference card for a book.

```
Jones, P.
1995

Spiritual Distress and the Practical Response:
Theoretical Considerations and Counselling
Skills: Journal of Advanced Health Care, 12,
377-82.

Keywords: Spiritual, counselling, nursing

Comments: A discussion of the problems of
'dispiritedness'. Not necessarily a 'religious'
question but definitely a 'spiritual' one.
Comments on how counselling skills may be used.
```

Figure 5.1b Reference card for a journal.

COMPUTER DATABASES

Databases for computer come in two types: the fixed-form database and the free-form sort. I will discuss both as both have their advantages and disadvantages.

THE FIXED-FORM DATABASE

First, some definitions. A form, in database jargon is a single record. Thus an entry containing all the details of one book is called a form. Each form contains a number of **fields**. A field is a discrete unit of information. Thus the place where you put the author's name is a field. So is the place where you put the date. So is the place where you put the title and so on.

With a fixed-form database, you have to work out a number of things before you start to file away your references. First, you need to know **how many** fields you will have. Then, you need to know the **maximum length** of any given field. For example, a simple reference database might have the following fields (and I have numbered them so that you can see at a glance how many fields there are):

1. Surname and initials of author
2. Year of publication
3. Title
4. Publisher and place of publication
5. Keywords
6. Comments

For all of these fields, you will need to consider the **length** of those fields. You have to know this sort of information in advance of entering data. There is a problem here. It is tempting, at first, to play safe and make the fields as long as possible – just in case you get an author with a triple-barrelled name or a title that goes on forever. On the other hand, if you do this, you are likely to take up a lot of space on your hard disk. Also, databases with long fields take a long time to 'search' (or look up) and with some databases, the display on the screen may be affected by long fields. You need to think carefully, then about a reasonable length for each field. Here are some values that I have found useful. The numbers in each case refer to the number of **characters** that can be used in a field. A character is a number, figure or space.

1. Author (100)
2. Date (4)
3. Title (250)
4. Publisher (200)
5. Keywords (50)
6. Comments (250)

Why 250 for the longer fields? Many databases have an upper limit of 250 characters per field.

When you are designing your database, you may want to add additional fields. Here are some that you may want to consider:

7. Location (library, home, work, named person)
8. Date of this entry
9. Lent to

and so on.

Be careful, though. Do not make your database system too complicated. Simplicity is important here. If you make your database lengthy and complicated you will find yourself skipping many of the fields and end up with an incomplete database. As a rule, only record the information that you are going to need in the future.

Once you have settled on the layout, the fields and the field lengths, you are stuck with that format. While it is possible to change the format at a later date, it can be difficult. The best thing to do is to have a few trial runs at making database layouts. Then choose the one that looks and feels best.

Once you have worked out the layout of your forms and fields, you can begin to enter the data. You can put the references in any order for the program can order all your cards afterwards. Mostly, you will want them indexed, alphabetically, by author but you can choose other permutations. Also, you can ask the database to call up all the entries that contain a particular keyword. Thus, you can call up all the entries that contain the keyword COUNSELLING and browse through all the references that you have collected on that topic. Further, you can narrow your search, if you have a lot of references on a particular topic. If, for example, you have hundreds of references on GROUPS, you may want to limit your search to GROUPS, THERAPY. The database program will then call up only those references that are to do with group therapy rather than just groups.

Also, you might want to call up all of a particular author's works on a particular subject. An example of this would be calling up everything that you have by Carl Rogers on client-centred counselling. This would mean that the program would ignore anything that Rogers had written (and you had collected) on topics such as humanistic psychology or student-centred learning. The database program can be a very flexible way of working with your reference collection. I know that I would be very reluctant to go back to a card system. As always, **backup** your database files. If your hard disk crashes, it is likely that you will have lost all your hard-found references.

EXAMPLES OF FIXED-FORM DATABASE PROGRAMS

There are numerous commercial programs on the market. The larger ones include the following.

Access

This is a large and powerful database program from the makers of Word for Windows. It is, however, also one of the easiest to use. I used to use it for storing bibliographical references and still use it, at work, to store student records.

Dataease

This is a powerful, menu-driven and easy to use database that allows you considerable latitude in designing the data-input screen.

dBase

Until fairly recently, this was probably the most famous database program. Currently it is in its dBase IV version. Not very easy to use, dBase may be too complicated for use as a reference database but it is ideal for storing research data.

Paradox

Powerful and yet easy to use: hence the name. The two features do not usually go hand in hand. I have known a number of people who use this database as a referencing system.

R:Base and R:Base Personal

Another powerful, dBase type database system. The Personal version is cut-down but still very usable and suitable for a referencing system.

Q and A Write

This is a very straightforward program that is a pleasure to use. I have found it useful for storing the details of students on a university course that I run and would probably use it to store references if I did not use a free-form system already (see below).

These programs vary in price and complexity. Remember that you ideally want something that is simple to use and to 'query'. (Database programmers talk about 'querying the database', meaning 'looking something up'.) You may well find that one of the shareware programs is just what you need. The concept of shareware was discussed in a previous chapter. Essentially, you pay a nominal amount to receive the program from a dealer. You then have between 30 and 90 days to review the program. If you continue to use it you are morally bound to send off a registration fee. This is usually a modest amount and for it you receive an updated version of the program and a detailed handbook about the work. Here are some useful shareware database programs that you may want to consider.

Vault

Vault is a Windows program that stores information as an outline. It helps you to organize information into categories and subcategories that you specify. You can also delete or create categories at any time. Vault's search command finds the information you need instantly and you can also browse through your outline by expanding and collapsing items. You can also print items from the program and, overall, it is a very flexible way of structuring and working with notes. This is a very 'simple' program to use but one that is also very useful. Any writer who needs to keep lots of notes in a readily accessible format is likely to find it useful.

Dream

Dream stands for Data Retrieval Entry And Management. It is a menu-driven database program that allows for three levels of data protection. It has on-line help and a tutorial system built in.

EFMS

Shareware writers seem to like acronyms. This name stands for Everyone's File Management System. It was designed to make data management simple. It provides efficient storage and quick retrieval for a wide variety of data and also allows you to paint your own screen.

File Express

This is possibly the easiest of all the database programs to set up and use. It is a simple program but one that can easily be used to store and retrieve references. Highly recommended.

Findex 3X5

This is a very simple program that works on a similar basis to the card system outlined above. Thus the name – 3X5 – refers to the size of small index cards. It is simple to use and to search.

Flexbase

Flexbase is a menu-driven data management system with context sensitive help. It was originally marketed as a commercial program but is now available as shareware.

Infobase

This is an integrated database program, form generator and mail-merge package. It is able to store up to 65 000 records, depending on the size of your hard disk.

Papers

This is a program that was specially designed for storing references. It has pre-prepared formats for papers and books and will recall your references easily and in a particular format. As we have noted elsewhere in this book, it is important to keep some form of recording system for bibliographical references and this is a useful program for doing that.

PC File

This is probably the best known of all the shareware database programs and easily comparable to many of the commercial offerings. I used it for a long time to store my references and found it easy to work with.

Zephyr

This is probably the most powerful of all the shareware programs. I found it a little slow to run on my computer and quite difficult to get to grips with. If you are prepared to invest a little time, it is likely to be the most universally useful database program at a very low price. Highly recommended.

If you are attracted to the fixed-form database start by sending away for a couple of shareware programs (perhaps File Express and PC File). This will cost you about £20 for the disks and the handling charges. Try these out. If you like one of them, stick to it. If not, consider moving into the commercial market and explore some of those programs. Remember, though, that you want to be able to access your references quickly and easily so do not go for anything too complicated.

FREE-FORM DATABASES

The free-form database does not use concepts such as fields and field length. With the free-form database, you simply open up a form, type in whatever it is you want to save, save the form and that is it. To look up an item of saved information, you simply key in one or two words that you know are in the form that you saved and the form comes on the screen. You are not limited by the format in which you enter data. You can put the author's name, followed by the title, followed by the date or you can start with a quotation and follow it with the bibliographic reference. The format really does not matter. All that matters is that you remember a word or two that occurs in the form that you have written. The free-form database program is rather like being able to collect together all sorts of different notes and pieces of paper and then being able to pull out the relevant ones whenever you want. I find the free-form approach much more liberating for storing bibliographic details. Figure 5.2 gives two examples of two forms from a free-form system. Note that both are in a very different format but that both can happily co-exist in the same database.

Davies, P. (1994) <u>Counselling Skills for Carers</u>, 2nd edn, Chapman & Hall, London.

This contains a number of chapters on counselling theory and reviews different approaches to counselling. It does not only address client-centred counselling but considers other types too.

I have lent my copy of this to David Jones. Remember to ring him about this.

His address is:

David Jones,
35 Blakemore Cottages
Denfield,
Herts
CF4 3RT

Also, consider the books by Rogers when it comes to writing up the counselling research project.

Keywords: Counselling, humanistic psychology, psychoanalysis, behavioural psychology.

This is a list of some of the books on COUNSELLING that may be helpful. Remember to look in Cardiff Central Library, too. They have a lot of useful books.

Baruth, L. G. (1987) <u>An Introduction to the Counselling Profession</u>, Prentice Hall, Englewood Cliffs, New Jersey

Bolger, A. W. (ed.) (1982) <u>Counselling in Britain: a reader</u>, Batsford Academic, London

Dryden, W., Charles-Edwards and Woolfe, R. (1989) <u>Handbook of Counselling in Britain</u>, Routledge

Figure 5.2 Examples of forms from a free-form system.

There are various free-form database programs available and these are three useful ones.

Memory Mate

This is available as a shareware program, when it is know as Instant Recall. It is very easy to set up and use and can be used as a Terminate and Stay Resident (or 'pop-up') program. You can use it over the top of your word processor and cut and paste references from it into the document you are working in. This is a DOS program that does not run, directly, under Windows.

Info Select

This is another excellent memory-resident free-form database program. Information is stored in individual windows that you can browse through, edit, search, select and form lists at will. When you begin the first few letters of a word, if that word appears somewhere in the database, you will be taken straight to that entry. Information can be keyed in or transferred in from your word processor. This is a highly recommended database program. It is a Windows program but it is also available in a DOS version.

Idealist

This is another excellent program that runs under Windows. It can be used for a whole range of things from storing bibliographical references to helping in the analysis of interview and other qualitative data. This is the program that I currently use to store my bibliographical references. It is a Windows program.

MAINTAINING YOUR DATABASE

Whether you use the fixed-form database or the free-form database, a few basic rules apply to maintenance. First, always make sure you backup your database files to floppies once you have finished entering new data. Second, get to know the program well. Learn how to index and how to transfer data from your database to your word processors and vice versa. Be careful to plan your database layout before you begin to use it. The best place to start is with pen and paper. Try a few layouts on paper before you experiment with the program itself. Databases are personal things, rather in the way that word processors are. Do not use a particular one just because someone has recommended it to you. Try to review a few before making a final decision and then be prepared to change your mind.

Initially, I worked with a word-processing file full of references. This was a straightforward system until the file got rather large. With this system, you simple list your references, in alphabetical order, in an ordinary word-processing file, like this:

Bradbury, R. (1990) *Zen in the Art of Writing: Essays on Creativity*, Joshua Odell editions, Capra Press, Santa Barbara, California.

Gunning, R. (1968) *The Technique of Clear Writing*, 2nd edn, McGraw- Hill, London.

Jourard, S. (1971) *Self-Disclosure: an Experimental Analysis of the Transparent Self*, Wiley, New York.

Larson, M. (1986) *Literary Agents: How to Get and Work with the Right One for You*, Writer's Digest Books, Cincinnati, Ohio.
Scott Fitzgerald, F. (1985) *Afternoon of an Author.* In L. W. Phillips (ed.), *F. Scott Fitzgerald on Writing*, Scribner, New York.
Wright Mills, C. (1959) *The Sociological Imagination*, Oxford University Press, Oxford.

You are then free to cut and paste references into papers and articles that you write. If your word processor has an automatic sorting function, you can enter the references into the file in any order. Then you ask the word processor to sort, alphabetically.

I used this system for a couple of years. I would call up the reference file every time I wrote a paper and kept it on the 'second screen'. That meant that I could easily switch between the paper I was writing and the reference file. Once this file became too big, I looked at a variety of simple database programs and finally settled on Idealist.

DATA PROTECTION ACT

If you keep details about other people, on disk, you must register under the Data Protection Act. There are eight general principles behind the act. These are as follows.

- Personal data must be collected and used fairly without deceiving those concerned.
- Personal data must be registered under the Act.
- If you are going to pass on personal data to other people you must state this when you register.
- You should not keep more personal data than you need.
- You have to try to make sure that personal data is accurate and up to date.
- You should not keep personal data for longer than you need to.
- If you hold personal data about somebody, they have the right to know what it is and to check that it is accurate.
- You have to try to make sure that personal data is not changed, destroyed or disclosed without authorization. (Branscombe, 1991)

To register under the act cost £75 in 1991 and lasts for three years. Forms can be obtained from the Registrar's office (02625 535777). The information you will require will include the following:

- the personal data that you are recording;
- what you use the data for;
- where you get this information from;
- who you may want to disclose the information to;
- any overseas countries where you may want to send the information.

You do not have to register under the act if you are merely keeping a personal address book, nor do you have to register if you keep a list of the members of a club of society. You should check with employees whether or not you are covered by the Act if you use your own database systems to record details of students on courses. You must consider, too, whether or not you need to register if you record personal details about people for a research project. Clearly, you do not have to register in order to maintain databases of non-personal details such as bibliographies.

Educational writing | 6

To write simply is as difficult as to be good.

Somerset Maugham

Most lecturers and educationalists have to write. For university and college lecturers, writing is sometimes part of the job. They are required to contribute articles and books as part of their contribution to the literature. The last two chapters of this book are concerned, specifically, with writing articles and books. The aim of this chapter is to explore elements of writing as it applies to preparing educational materials.

The sort of writing that has to be done by a teacher or lecturer will include the following:

- preparation of overhead transparencies;
- preparation of handouts;
- writing of course material;
- writing of curriculum documents;
- preparing notes for a presentation or conference;
- writing letters, memos and faxes;
- sending e-mail messages.

OVERHEAD TRANSPARENCIES

Overhead transparencies (OHPs) are widely used by teachers and lecturers. They are a means of conveying headings and specific information to large groups of people. They also take the spotlight off the teacher or lecturer and allow her to concentrate on good delivery.

These days, most laser printers or photocopiers can produce print onto acetate sheets. If your laser or dot matrix printer cannot, your photocopier is likely to. Now you have no excuse for scrappy, handwritten OHPs. Instead, you can print out single sheets of text which you then photocopy onto acetates, making enlargements as necessary. Certain key principles apply to the preparation of material for OHPs:

- keep them simple
- use clear and straightforward graphics to illustrate a point, where possible;
- use only one or two fonts – no more;
- use only a few lines per sheet.

I once sat through the most boring lecture I can remember. The lecturer used a single sheet which was covered in writing. She slowly revealed a single line of text and took about ten minutes to talk through each item. You knew how much longer the lecture had to run by the amount of revelation she made. The lecture seemed to go on for ever.

Although the revelation technique is widely taught as a method of working through OHPs, I think that it has one big disadvantage. It reminds the students of how much is to come. Better, I think, to use one or two straightforward acetates that you reveal completely and then talk to. Do not have too many sheets. Almost as daunting as the sheet covered in writing that is gradually revealed is the ominous looking pile of acetates next to the projector that you **know** the lecturer is going to get through, come what may. Again, keep it short and simple. Use illustrations where ever possible. Try to make your presentations as professional as possible.

Some lecturers like to use slides. Again, make full use of these by taking photographs and showing these, interspersed with single slides containing words. Usually, slides with writing on have a blue background with white lettering. Try, if you can, to ring the changes and have different colour backgrounds. Also, consider combining either two slide projectors and two screens or the OHP machine and a slide machine. I have seen joint use of these contribute to a very effective presentation.

Don't overuse slides. Use perhaps five or six. Any more and the presentation gets to be reminiscent of those awful evenings that you sometimes get invited to when a friend shows her holiday slides or photos. Most people overestimate other people's interest in a particular topic. Make sure, too, that your slides are of the highest quality and that all are set in the right position in the slide projector. Nothing upsets the lecturer and amuses an audience quite as much as an upside-down slide. When you show the slide, after a quick glance to see that it is both up the right way and also the right slide, talk to the audience and not to the slide. Allow people a little time to stare at the slide and do not offer any important information during the first 30 seconds of slide display. Try, if you can, to use the slides and OHP material to surprise and delight the audience. Boring slides can do nothing to stimulate an audience and nothing to improve the quality of your presentation.

Use a graphics programme to produce clear printed sheets, perhaps containing three or four lines, in a single font.

Whatever you do, make sure that all your visual aids are professionally prepared. Become familiar with what your graphics program can use and use it minimally. That is to say that you should not become over ambitious. You can always tell the amateur who has just acquired a graphics package: her OHPs are covered with familiar graphics symbols from well-known graphics programs. Often, butterflies, balloons or buildings feature strongly in such presentations.

PREPARATION OF HANDOUTS

Many of the principles of OHP preparation apply to handouts. Keep them simple and use only one or two fonts in their preparation. Make sure that all photocopies are clearly printed and completely readable.

Conventional teaching wisdom has it that you should not give out handouts during a lecture but you should give them out at the end. This is to stop the distraction of the pile of papers being handed round the room. It is also to stop people reading the handouts instead of listening to you. In practice, I find it useful to do one-page handouts that contain broad headings and to give those out. If these pages are clearly numbered, they stop the need for students to jot down notes continually as you are speaking and they have a permanent aide memoir of your lecture. Again, if you prepare such handouts carefully and professionally, it reflects well on you as a lecturer. Scrappy or unclear handouts also reflect on you.

Go easy with book lists. The temptation is to hand out three or four page lists of books. Few people read through such lists and I suspect that few lecturers have read all the books on their lists. Anyone, really, can compile huge bibliographies fairly easily. Instead, consider one-page book lists, containing, perhaps, six or seven titles that constitute **essential** reading. Then offer yourself as a resource for the keen student who wants advice about further reading.

WRITING OF COURSE MATERIALS

Course materials can range from reading lists and handouts to study guides for students. Try to make these as professional as possible. Use a desktop publishing program to help you with the layout and stick to one or two fonts. Try to keep a unifying theme running through all your presentations and consider having the course book that you prepare professionally printed. Many printers now can print directly from your disk. If you cannot afford to do this, laser print the main copy and make sure that subsequent photocopies are clear and readable.

Consider how you will bind course material. It is possible to buy simple binders fairly cheaply or you may want to invest in a professional binding machine. Spiral and comb binding are falling out of fashion and tend to offer a less than professional finish. Avoid splashy graphics on the front cover of your course books and keep the whole presentation simple. Make sure that there are page numbers on each page but avoid cluttered headers and footers.

Think about what might go into a course book that will tell your students all they know about your course. Here are some sections that you may want to consider:

- front sheet with title of the course and name of course leader;
- short paragraph on a single page that welcomes the student to the course book;
- contents page;
- aims of the course;
- educational philosophy;
- teaching and learning methods used;
- assessments, including details of all essays, project work and examinations;
- content: week by week and session by session;
- reading list;
- biographical details of teachers on the course;
- appendix: how to reference an essay: the Harvard or Vancouver method;
- index.

Most students appreciate a clear handbook to a course. It can offer them milestones to work towards and make the whole thing seem manageable. Also, it seems reasonable to give students prior notice of how they will be assessed. The Americans seem to be much better at this sort of thing that people in the UK. In many American colleges, students are **sold** the course handbook. It seems unlikely that this will happen in the UK – at least, not within the next six months.

The index may seem to be something of a problem. If you are working in one of the larger word processors such as WordPerfect, you can use the program to produce a detailed index of the document. Indexes always improve the quality of longer documents and you are advised to consider their use in your course handbook.

WRITING OF CURRICULUM DOCUMENTS

Some lecturers and teachers have to plan courses. Course planning seems to be a full-time job for many people these days. Some lecturers are employed just for this task. Again, the more clearly you can plan and design any material you send out to curriculum working groups the better. Also, a professional package that offers the whole of your curriculum is more likely to help in the validation process than a scrappy-looking one. Try not to make these sorts of documents too long. Although some validation boards lay down strict guidelines for the preparation of such material, many do not. If you have not been given guidelines, do not assume that you have to produce 500 page tomes. No one wants to read them and the validation board are unlikely to stay up all night to read them through. Write documents that people read. This seems an obvious statement but it is not. I am sure that many people write curricula with no idea of the reader in mind. Most readers of curricula are like you or me. We will read them if we have to and are paid to but we will not read them for pleasure. Keep your validators in a good mood, keep their reading down to a minimum.

Make full use of simple tables and figures but don't overload them with figures. If you use graphs, don't forget to label the axes and to tell the reader what they are looking at. Avoid complicated forms of bar charts that offer over-lays and multiple graphs and charts. They may be thought to look impressive but no one wants to struggle to understand them. Many people will ignore them all together.

Consider having the final curriculum document professionally bound. Most university and college printers can do this quite cheaply. Avoid reproducing photocopies of the college crest. If you can, see if the university or college printer has the original printing block that was used to print crests on other documents and ask him if he can use it on yours. Otherwise, keep the crest off altogether and use clear lettering instead. Avoid any sort of fancy borders or scrolls and – particularly – avoid the use of clip-art illustrations. Read through the whole document before it is bound and check for typographical errors (or 'typos' as they are known in the publishing world). Pedantic validation board members enjoy picking up course designers on their spelling and grammatical errors.

PREPARING NOTES

Many lecturers have to give papers at conferences. Many are terrified at the thought and many are not very good at it because they do not prepare sufficiently.

To read from notes or not to? Not to, as a rule. If at all possible, avoid reading directly from a script or straight from notes. If **you** can read what you have to say, so can your audience. If all you are doing is standing up and reading what you would normally publish in a journal, do the latter. Go away and write your journal paper. While you may not want to do without notes altogether (and few do), you want to try to keep your notes to key issues and an overall outline structure.

The most frequently used method of using notes at a presentation is that of holding a bunch of index cards in your hand, each of which contains notes linked to one of your three or four points. These have advantages and disadvantages. The advantages are that they are easy to hold and to refer to. You can hold your hands up fairly high and this tends to encourage you to speak out to your audience rather than down to your notes. On the other hand, small cards can be dropped. Once dropped, you have the unenviable (but fascinating to the audience in a morbid sort of way) task of picking them up and rearranging them. Just in case, it is best to number your cards with fairly large numbers so that your nervous hands can reorder them in a crisis.

It is usually best to link your cards with your visual presentations. As is noted in the next section, backing up what you say with things that the audience can look at pays distinct dividends. Usually, you can link one card with one visual aid. In this way, you don't have to carry out too many operations at once. Be sure, though, to number both your cards **and** your visual aids clearly. Visual aids can also be dropped or get out of order. If both the card and the aid bear the same number, you are less likely to run into problems.

The alternative to cards is to use a computer-generated set of notes. If you use this method, you need to have them typed with double spacing, so that you can read them easily as you glance down. Also, it is useful to make full use of coloured 'outlining' pens. Careful colour coding can show you where you are in relation to your main three or four points: each point can be outlined in a different colour and that colour code can be carried through to your visual aids. The big disadvantage of the typed sheets is that you are likely to get carried away with looking at them.

There is some comfort to be had from holding a large bunch of papers. Often, that comfort takes over and the speaker using them, stares down at them throughout the presentation: sometimes from fear of losing place. Think, too, about whether or not you staple the sheets together. The advantage of this approach is that you can hold the whole set of pages together, with less fear of dropping them. On the other hand, if you find yourself with a large lectern in front of you, unstapled sheets can more easily be turned over. I have been known to adopt the 'belt-and-braces' approach and take two sets of notes with me to a conference: one stapled and the other not.

If your confidence really leaves you and you decide that you **must** read from notes, consider the way that you write out those notes. Rather than just typing out a 'script', write out what you say in the way that you say it. Figure 6.1 illustrates this. The piece is laid out in such a way that it makes it very clear where you pause and where you take a breath. The idea is that each line contains one phrase. Work carefully through your notes and break them up in this way. This will save you 'fluffing' lines and save you having to re-read what you have said. It must be stressed, however, that reading direct from a paper is the last resort. If you can, avoid it.

One of the best ways of preparing this sort of paper is on a computer, using a word processor. It is possible, in some programs, to set up 'macros' or shorthand routines that operate 'sentence-busting' functions. Such macros split the whole of your paper up into sentences and put each sentence on a separate line. WordPerfect is one such word-processing program. It is possible with this word processor, not only to sentence-bust but also to reverse the process and put the paper back together again. In this way, you are able to prepare the paper that you use for your presentation and the more usual copies of the paper for wider distribution. Be careful, though: splitting the paper into sentences is not **all** that

Conference Paper: Change and the Health Professional
1. Many health professionals are having to think carefully about how change is affecting their organization.
2. Many are experiencing anxiety about the <u>rate</u> of change.
3. Writers on the topic are not always helpful here.
4. All seem to stress that change is accelerating.
5. This morning, I want to challenge that view.
6. The question is:Is the rate of change <u>really</u> increasing?
7. Think about your own workplace.
8. What changes have <u>you</u> seen?
9. Major ones?
10. Or have you experienced a slow trickle of minor changes?
11. If change <u>is</u> occurring, what difference does it make?
12. People as resilient and able to cope
13. Defence mechanisms
14. What the research tells us
15. Concluding comment

Figure 6.1 Example of notes for a conference paper.

is involved. You also need to go through the piece and underline or accent certain words so that you know exactly when to emphasize your points. Notice, too, that the piece, above, is not strictly grammatical.

You may want to consider the use of rhetorical questions that 'sound' right, when you speak but would not normally be acceptable in a written paper. Again, this is further fuel for the argument that you should try to avoid reading directly from a script. On the other hand, if you are giving a lot of very detailed information and that information must be exactly right, then reading may be your only option. Consider, for example, newsreaders on the television. No one would expect **them** to extemporize with the help of cue cards.

CURRICULUM VITAE

The other sort of educational writing that many lecturers and educationalists have to write or advise other people about is writing a curriculum vitae. The curriculum vitae is just that: a 'life curriculum' or description of your life to date. Think carefully about what you put in it. It is usually a good idea to keep a copy of your CV in your possession at all times and to update it regularly. That way, when you apply for a job, there is no problem in remembering what you have and have not done. If you use a computer and word processor, it is useful to keep your CV as a file and to add to the file as new things happen to you. You may want to keep a 'short version' that summarizes the essential parts of your personal history, as well as the full version. The short version can be a useful aid to filling in application forms and may be asked for during applications for jobs, grants or scholarships. It is also possible to write macros in a word-processing program to recall, quickly, your prepared CV.

CVs typically cover the following subject areas:

- name;
- address;
- work address;
- date of birth;
- age;
- marital status;
- place of birth;
- nationality;
- current post;
- secondary, professional and higher education;
- other professional training (short courses, management courses etc.);
- professional employment;
- summary of responsibilities in present post;
- committee membership;
- other professional activities (membership of unions, clubs, associations, editorial boards, external examining etc.);
- other activities (governorship of schools, membership of other organizations etc.);
- miscellaneous section (driving licence, word-processing skills etc.);
- research;
- conference papers;
- publications (books, chapters in books, articles in refereed journals, articles in other journals).

You might not use all of these headings nor will they all be appropriate to everyone's CV but you should aim at making your CV as comprehensive as possible. Make sure that all of the dates are correct and that the spelling and layout are appropriate. At the end of the CV it is sometimes correct to include the names and addresses of two or three people who will write references for you. Make sure that you ask those people's permission to quote their names before you do so.

Make sure that you spend some time on the layout of your CV. Too many people spoil an otherwise excellent CV by one or other of two extremes. Some spoil the document by overuse of a desktop publishing program. Such people use coloured paper, lots of different size fonts and full use of banner headlines and so forth. They make their CV look more like a parish newsletter than a serious document of their lives. At the other extreme, some people type their CV on a battered typewriter with an old ribbon and an uneven typeface. Try for something in the middle. Laser print your CV but use only standard headings and subheadings. Use white paper only and try, above all things, to make the document look businesslike. It is, after all, a sales document.

Note that, nowadays, many word processors are supplied with a CV template or a method of formatting a CV to make it look professional and to standardize the layout.

Another sort of CV is one that concentrates on your achievements. In this type, you write out your life history in terms of your educational and professional posts and under each one you list the things that you achieved. An example of such an entry might be the following:

Lecturer in Health Visiting, University of Blackheath: 1979–1981.
During this period, I was course leader for the health visiting course. I rewrote the curriculum, advised on promotion and advertising and was able to recruit three times the number of students in 1980 than in the previous year.

WRITING LETTERS, MEMOS, FAXES AND E-MAIL

Most educators, like most managers, have to send a variety of letters, memos and faxes. Most people soon get the hang of wording such documents and, once again, the key features of simplicity and structure apply. There are also some conventions for laying out such documents. Figures 6.2–6.5 show the layout for e-mail, letters, memos and faxes.

Fashions in layout change. Currently, it is popular to use the 'block' paragraph layout for paragraphs in letters, memos and faxes. Also, it is usual to layout text 'ranged left'. That is to say that headings, addresses and so forth are lined up against the left margin rather than centred on the page or ranged to the right.

Bear in mind that if you are using a modern word processor, you can usually set up a template or a macro that will allow you to call up a 'blank' letter, memo or fax page and then simply 'fill in the blanks'. This approach is not only economical of time but it also helps you to maintain a consistent corporate image.

Note that memos don't usually need to be signed by the sender and may not need an envelope if they are being sent through an internal postal system. As a rule, they should be kept short: you want them to be **read**.

When writing faxes, it is often better to use a sans serif font for the body text of the fax – as shown in the example on page 94. A sans serif font tends to 'copy' better when passed through the two fax machines. Note that you can either use a cover page that is blank – except for the details of the person sending it and the

Dear Peter,
Do you have any details of the work of Peters and Davies on learning styles? I believe they developed a learning styles inventory some years ago but I can't find it.
Regards, David French, University of West London

. . . .

Dear David,
I found your learning styles inventory. It was published in a journal that only has a small circulation and I can understand why you missed it. Here is the reference:
Peters, D.A. and Davies, P. (1995) Measuring How People Learn: is it possible? New England Health Care Journal, 3, 4, 23-56.
A colleague in Florida has used the inventory. Do you want me to get her to contact you?
Regards, Peter Zander, University of Chicago.

. . . .

Dear Peter,
Thanks for the reference - I have tracked down the paper. That was useful. Yes, I would be delighted to hear from your colleague in Florida. Thanks again.
Regards, David

. . . .

Dear David French,
Peter Zander at the University of Chicago asked me to contact you. I hear that you are interested in using the Peters and Davies' learning styles inventory. I have used it with four groups of between 100-150 students and will send you a summary of my findings. Perhaps we could do some collaborative research on this?
Regards, Sally Henderson, Lecturer in Health Care Studies, University of Southern Florida, E-mail address sallyh@fla.edu

Figure 6.2 Example of e-mail dialogue.

person receiving it – as the first page of your fax or you can write your message straight onto the first page of the fax. It is often preferable to use a 'blank' cover page if you know that your fax contains sensitive information or if you that it may lie in a pile of other faxes at the organization to whom you are sending it.

Scotfield University College
23-45 Anderson Road
Scotfield
Surrey
SC1 N4T

Phone: 0243-342523

24th May 1996

Dr Sarah Jones
56 Petersfield Road
Langley
South Glamorgan
CF5 43L

Dear Sarah

Stress Reduction Teaching

Thank you your recent letter. I am glad that you were able to use the activities that I suggested. I have found them particularly useful when teaching small groups.

I hope that we will be able to keep in touch about these approaches to helping people with stress. I look forward to hearing from you again.

With best wishes,

Yours sincerely,

Dr Susan Brownloe
Director of Health Care Studies

Figure 6.3 Layout of a letter.

In these cases, the cover page serves to cover up the information contained in your fax.

As with all writing, it is important to make sure that memos, letters and faxes are clear and make use of simple language. The days of letters being written in a peculiar 'officialese' are largely over but it is still possible to find people writing, regularly, 'Please find the enclosed copy of the report' instead of the more straightforward: 'Here is a copy of the report.'

E-MAIL

The style of writing when sending and responding to e-mail is much less formal than is the case with letters, memos and faxes. E-mail communication is almost like a conversation. It is quite acceptable to write in note form when responding to e-mail. An example of a continuing 'correspondence' might look like Figure 6.2.

MEMO

To: Jane Johnson, Senior Health Lecturer, University
    College

From: Peter Barker, Lecturer, School of Occupational
      Therapy, University College

Date: 23.4.96

Re: Course Evaluation

Thank you for sending me the evaluation questionnaires. I have made copies of them and circulated
them to my colleagues. Once I have used the questionnaires with the students group, I will collate
the findings and send you the findings

Figure 6.4 Layout of a memo.

Scotfield University College
23-45 Anderson Road
Scotfield
Surrey
SC1 N4T

Fax Cover Sheet

DATE: 31 May 1995   **TIME:**   09:37

TO: Mr P. Jones   **PHONE:** 01243-342523
           Anderson Health College   **FAX:**   01243-353243
FROM: Dr A. Davies   **PHONE:** 01453-234525
           Scotfield University College   **FAX:**   01453-465463

RE: Interdisciplinary Health Teaching
CC: Mrs J. Arthurs, Personal Assistant

Number of pages including cover sheet: 1

Thank you for the curriculum document. I will take it to the curriculum planning
committee in this college, this afternoon. I will then contact you again with
further details of the next stage, directly after the meeting.
This is the name and address that you need in order to purchase copies of the
open learning materials that we discussed:

Peter Sharpe
Abacus Open Learning College
34 London Road
Abingail
Wiltshire
WV4 5D6 Phone: 01442-564364

Figure 6.5 Layout of a fax.

It should be noted that new messages on the e-mail will be prefaced by details of the sender, their e-mail address and the route by which the e-mail message travelled. These details are omitted in the example (Figure 6.2). Those details can run to many lines of screen print-out.

CONCLUSION

All educational writing is a form of communication. It is also part of the educational process. You should spend time planning out how you will use printed matter. After all, it is the format that most people use to learn a lot of what they know. Students will spend hours reading books and journal articles. Don't insult them by giving them poorly prepared handouts or course material. Do not upset them by offering them ill prepared OHPs during your lectures. Besides, planning and designing this sort of material can be interesting in and of itself. Read more about layout and printing. Particularly, learn the basic rules of layout and make them second nature. Then your own printed work will always look professional and will be appreciated by your students and your colleagues.

Writing essays

7

> Clear writers, like clear fountains, do not seem so deep as they are; the turbid look the most profound.
>
> Walter Savage Landor

If you are doing a course of some kind, that lasts longer than a week, you are likely to have to write essays. Essays are an almost universal form of assessment. While there are numerous titles for essays, there are some simple rules about writing that can be learned fairly easily. The aim of this chapter is to make your essay-writing easier. It has to be said, though, that some people like writing and write easily while others struggle to put pen to paper or fingers to keyboard. Whether you find it pleasure or pain, the keynote, once again, is **structure**. If you can get the structure right you are likely to find the writing easier. This applies if this is your first or 31st essay. No one should sit down and begin to write the first line of an essay without prior planning.

The planning stages of an essay are as follows:

- reading the question;
- underlining key words;
- brainstorming;
- writing the essay outline;
- collecting information.

READING THE QUESTION

This would seem to be a straightforward requirement. Many people tend to write the essay they **think** should be written rather than the one that is asked for. Some people have a 'standard' essay that is almost automatically written whenever key words are seen. For example, an essay about counselling skills in helping bereaved people may cause some people to write everything they know about counselling. This is not the point at all. It is vital to answer the question. This can only happen if you read the question carefully and re-read it.

UNDERLINING THE KEY WORDS

Once you have read the question, underline the key words. This is not as simple as it sounds. Some people find when they first do this that they underline almost all of the words in the essay title. Here is a sample question to work on:

Critically evaluate the use of therapy groups in a specific health care setting.

Read through the title two or three times and then underline the key words. The underlining that I did was as follows:

Critically evaluate the use of *therapy groups* in a *specific health care setting.*

Now consider what the essay is asking you to do. First, you are asked to **critically evaluate** something. Not describe it. Not define it but critically evaluate it. Think carefully about what that means. Then, you are given the subject of that critical evaluation: **therapy groups**. This means that you have to be clear about what therapy groups might be and you will need to say this in your essay. Finally, you are asked to do all of this within a **specific health care setting**. As no other details are given, it can be taken as read that you can choose the health care setting. Make sure that you do. Make sure that you tell the reader what setting you have chosen. All of this must happen before you move on to the next stage of brainstorming.

BRAINSTORMING

Most people are fairly familiar with the process of brainstorming and it is only briefly described here. It is noteworthy that while brainstorming tends to be taught in UK schools and colleges, formal outlining of essays does not. In Canada and the USA, outlining is taught at junior school level. Perhaps we need to give it more attention in this country. It can make all the difference in essay writing.

Brainstorming involves giving the imagination free rein around the topic in hand. Having read the question and having identified what the question is about, the brainstorming phase is concerned with your jotting down on a piece of paper all the words or associations that you can think of related to the question. These should be written down in any order and **everything** is permitted. Make no attempt to filter out any words of phrases and do not work at 'ordering' at this stage. The dafter ideas often spark of useful ones. Here is an example of some of the things that I 'brainstormed' around the above question:

- group therapy
- gestalt therapy

- group facilitation
- health care setting: acute psychiatric unit
- psychiatrist
- psychologist
- who runs the group?
- research into groups?
- do groups work?
- my wife doesn't like groups much
- types of group facilitation
- does therapy work?
- J. Masson: *Beyond Therapy*
- references for this essay?
- I like group work
- I like running groups
- I don't enjoy being a member so much
- are groups about power?
- how do you evaluate groups?
- what is a group?
- offer clear definitions at the start of your essay
- who is this essay for?
- groups or counselling: which is best?
- training

This process should carry on for as long as you can still make associations around the title of the essay. The process may last for five minutes or it may last for fifteen. Do not leave any thoughts out and allow yourself to muse a little.

Next, work through the list and cross out any obviously inappropriate words or phrases. In the above list, I think I would cross out 'I don't like being a member so much' and 'groups or counselling: which is best'. Both have relevance for the essay in that they reminded me about my own bias in group work and about counselling – related but not directly relevant issues. The last point also reminded me of a book by Richard Nelson Jones in which he discusses 'group counselling'. However, neither of those two phrases seem directly related to the topic in hand.

The next stage is to group together the various issues into some sort of order. This is often best done under a series of headings. The headings that seem to emerge from the above list would include:

- the context (the setting)
- definitions
- problems of evaluation
- issues in running therapy groups

From this initial grouping together, the structure of a possible essay begins to emerge and it is possible to begin to draw up an outline. An outline is what it says: the headings and subheadings of your essay. An outline for the above essay might look like this:

1. Introduction

    1.   **What this essay is about**

    2.   **Definitions**
        1. Therapy groups
        2. Health care setting
        3. Evaluation

    3.   **Health care setting**
        1. Acute psychiatric unit
        2. Brief description
        3. Uses of therapy groups in this setting

    4.   **Evaluating groups**
        1. Short review of the research
        2. Methods of evaluating groups

    5.   **Critical issues**
        1. Lack of specific research
        2. Difficulty in deciding whether or not group work is effective in psychiatry
        3. Tendency of some practitioners to prefer group work

    6.   **Summary**
        1. Summing up: review of the main points
        2. Directions for future work
        3. Conclusions

    7.   **References**

Once the outline is completed, it is important to check back to the question and to the brainstorming to check that the outline is for an essay that answers the question. Read through the above outline and be critical of it yourself. Is it likely to answer the question? Does it look as though key issues may be left out? How does it compare to an essay that **you** might write on the topic? Essays are bound to reflect the view of the person who writes them. They will also vary in 'depth' according to the course they are being written on. You would not necessarily expect a detailed, analytical and researched-based paper on a pre-training course. You would expect such a paper on a masters degree course.

Make sure that you are writing the right sort of essay for the course you are working on. If you are unsure of the level, ask to see an example essay. Most lecturers are able to show you something of this sort if they are pushed, although some are hedgy about the issue.

COLLECTING INFORMATION

Using the outline, you can collect all the information you need to write your essay. Often, this will involve the library. It will mean your collecting 'references': details of books and papers related to the topic in your essay. You can get this information in a number of ways. The following is a list of some of those ways.

- By browsing through the library shelves. This can be time-consuming but can turn up some surprises. It can produce serendipitous findings: surprising and pleasant. It can also waste a lot of time.
- By working through the books that you already have on the topic and referring to the books that have been used by the writer. If you were writing an essay on writing, for example, you could turn to the bibliography section of this book to find more references.
- By using library bibliographies. These are large volumes in the library that list all recent publications in a given field. They often list an abstract of a particular book or paper, too.
- By using CD-ROM. This is a compact-disc, computerized system of bibliographic storage. It is the most efficient way of finding references. You can print out lists of the references you need, filter huge lists of references down to more specific lists. You can also download your reference lists onto floppy disk for use later on.

Once you have got your references together, you need to record them in the format described in the earlier chapter. Then, you need to find the books and papers and read them.

WRITING THE ESSAY

All that remains is to write the essay. Using the outline, work through each of the headings and follow the plan. Make sure that you **only** write about the issues under the particular heading. Be careful that you do not get carried away and write everything down under one heading.

Use the headings from your proposal as headings in the essay. Although opinions differ about whether or not headings should be used in essays, the trend towards their use seems to have increased. On the whole, they tend to lend structure to the essay and offer 'signposts' to the reader. More traditional lecturers may ask that you avoid using them.

Also a matter of debate is whether or not you should highlight the main points of your essay in your introduction. An example of such an introduction might be:

> Evaluation of **any** psychological therapy is likely to be difficult. The question of the efficacy of group therapy has been the subject of considerable debate but not of very much research. This paper opens with definitions of the terms used in it. The health care setting is then defined. The paper continues with a critical debate of the issue of evaluating group therapy in that context.

Despite the rather prosaic tone of this opening paragraph, it does help to guide the reader to what is going to be in the essay. Likewise, a similar paragraph at the end of the essay helps to draw together the main threads and to highlight the important issues. Some, however, feel that both are redundant. Some academics prefer a more direct style that entails getting straight into the meat of the essay. Find out from the person who has set your essay which approach applies.

REFERENCES

Use references carefully in your essay. Never use them just to impress. In a sense, of course, this is a slightly pompous statement: you are **trying** to impress when you write your essay. References, though, should indicate that you are aware of the source of particular ideas, thoughts, research and so forth. You should not use them as cake decorations to brighten up your essay. Nor should you quote directly from text unless you feel that you cannot possibly paraphrase what the other writer has written. Direct quotations should be gems. Also, it is best to gather your references together at the ends of sentences rather than scattering them throughout. Consider, for example, this clumsy sentence:

> Rogers (1967), however, took issue with Buber (1952) over the question of evil: with May (1956) Buber had challenged Rogers' apparent failure to address what has been called 'the problem of evil' (Brown, 1967; Davidson, 1984).

A tidier and more easily read sentence might be:

> Rogers was sometimes accused of ignoring the question of evil. (Buber, 1952; May, 1956).

Remember, too, to pay attention to the way that you format references in your essay. In the next paragraphs, we consider the Harvard and Vancouver methods of references. Both are frequently used in academic essays and in journal papers. Again, it is essential to check with your lecturer about the style of referencing that you are to use.

THE HARVARD SYSTEM OF REFERENCING

The Harvard system of referencing is the one in which the name of the author and the date of publication appear in the body of the text and the full reference is listed at the end. Here is an example of the end of a paper in which the system has been used:

> The writer has discussed the question of whether or not all clients should attend group therapy sessions in another paper (Brown, 1987). Other writers have also discussed this issue, most notably Davis (1989) and Anderson (1990, 1991).

> *References*
> Anderson, P. (1990) Group Therapy for In Patients. *British Journal of Group Work,* **2**(4), 34–46.
> Anderson, P. (1991) *Working with Groups*, Heinemann, Oxford.
> Brown, D. (1987) Does Group Work Make a Difference? *Nursing Times,* **3**(5), 67–8.
> Davis, L. (1989) *Against Groups*, Pan, London.

The points that you need to pay close attention to with the Harvard system of referencing are these:

- Only the author's surname and the date of publication appear in the body of the text.
- In the reference list at the end of the essay, references are listed alphabetically, by author.
- If an author has two publications in the same year and both are referred to, one is called a and the other b (e.g. Brown 1989a, 1989b) Full references are listed at the end, noting, correctly, reference a and reference b.
- In the reference list, the following are always listed and in this order: author's surname, author's initials, date of publication, title, publisher, place of publication. This is true when the publication is a book. For journal references, the order is as follows: author's surname, author's initials, date of publication, title of journal, volume number, edition number, pages. In the list, book titles are underlined or italicized. With references to journal papers, the name of the journal is underlined. It is important to get this right.

SOME VARIANTS OF THE BASIC HARVARD SYSTEM

The basic Harvard system, then, involves the quotation of a surname and date, in brackets, in the main body of the text, with a full list of the references used, alphabetically by author, at the end of the text. There is a range of variations of this method and some of these are now described. These should be used as guidelines: there are sometimes 'local' variations in colleges and departments: personal preferences of lecturers and journal editors sometimes mean that approaches **other** than the ones listed here are used. Overall, the really important issue is that you are **consistent** in the way that you use references.

Works having two or three authors

Where a book or paper has two or three authors, these should be listed, in the order they appear in the original publication, in parentheses with the date, in the text, e.g. (Brown, Smith and Jones, 1993).

Works having more than three authors

Where a book or paper has more than three authors, the first should be quoted, followed by '*et al.*' in parentheses, before the date, e.g. (Davies *et al.*, 1995). In the list of references, at the back of the paper, **all** authors should be quoted in full. Some authorities prefer the use of '*et al.*' for books and papers that have more than two authors while others prefer to use it where there are two or more.

When a work has a corporate author

When a book or paper has no individual's name offered as author, it is usual to quote the **organization's** name as the author, e.g. (British Association of Health Workers, 1994). An alternative is to **abbreviate** the organization when you cite the reference the first time and, subsequently, to use that abbreviation. Example:

> First citation: This point was developed in a report on handwashing in the workplace (British Association of Health Workers (BAHW), 1994).

> Second and subsequent citations: The issue of washing hands both before and after handling food has been dealt with elsewhere (BAHW, 1994).

When an author has published more than one book or paper in the same year

It is sometimes necessary to quote various papers, by the same author, published in the same year. In this case, it is usual to designate each an 'a', 'b', 'c' and so on, e.g. (James, 1992a; 1992b, 1992c). In the reference list, these are written out in full, complete with the appropriate letter after the date.

When a reference is to a chapter in a book edited by another author

It is quite often necessary to quote a chapter (by one author) in a book edited by another. Here, the name of the author of the **chapter** is cited in brackets, with the date. In the reference list, full details of both the chapter and the book are written out. Here is an example of both the reference in the text and the listing in the reference list.

> Various writers have discussed the question of health care funding in areas where there is a large population of elderly people. Davies (1994) has suggested that local funding is rarely adequate.

> Davies, P. D. (1994) Local Funding of Health Care. In P. Brown and T. Smith, *The Economics of Local Health Care*, Chapman & Hall, London.

When one author is quoted by another

Sometimes, it is impossible to go back to primary sources and to find out what an author wrote, directly. In this case, it becomes necessary to use **another** author's quoting of the original author. Imagine, for example, that you have picked up a book called *Counselling in the Health Services* by an author called David Smith, published in 1995. In this book, Smith writes as follows:

> The concept of empathy is a difficult one. We probably all know what if feels like to be understood but being totally understood is another matter. Brown writes about it as follows:

> No single person can ever fully understand another. The idea that empathy is something that can be taught is fraught with problems. We do not get 'taught' to empathize. Instead, we learn it through the process of growing up with other people. (Brown, 1993)

If you wanted to use this information about Brown in your **own** work, you would have to quote it as follows:

> Brown (cited by Smith, 1995) suggests that we probably cannot be **taught** to empathize but have to learn it through the process of living alongside others.

In the reference list, you would quote the Smith book as follows:

> Smith, D. (1995) *Counselling in the Health Services*, Butterworth-Heinemann, Oxford.

This is a rather complicated issue. Wherever possible, it is best to **avoid** this sort of citation. Wherever possible, go back to the original source of the information. In this case, you would try to find Brown's book and work directly from that. It is certainly not good practice to rely on one or two textbooks and to use lots of 'cited by' references by pulling out information from these one or two sources.

When two authors have the same surname

When two different authors, with the same name, are referred to in a paper or manuscript, it is important to include their **initials** so that the reader can be sure

about to which one you are referring, e.g.

> I. J. Davies (1994) discusses a range of issues to do with GP practice and the use of antibiotics. In another paper, P. D. Davies (1994) indentifies some of the more common side effects of the broad-spectrum antibiotics.

Personal communications

Personal communications may include letters, memos, telephone conversations and face-to-face conversations. Generally, it is not good practice to cite personal communications in papers and manuscripts but sometimes this is the only way of identifying a source of information. When 'personal communication' is cited, the reference is **only** placed in the body of the text and not included in the reference list at the end of the document. It is usual to offer the inititals and surname of the other person, along with the full date, e.g.

> For some, it is important to help depressed patients to externalize agression by forcing the person into a heated debate or argument. (J. Richards, personal communication, 12 May 1996)

It is important to learn the correct format for the Harvard referencing system. Once learned, it becomes second nature in the using. Also, many published books and journals use the system so you will quickly come to recognize its use. Until recently, it has been the most popular form of referencing system. The Vancouver system seems to be catching it up.

THE VANCOUVER SYSTEM OF REFERENCING

In the Vancouver system, a series of numbers is used to indicate that a reference is being used. Those references are then listed at the end of the paper, in numerical order, as those numbers appeared in the text. The above example, written with the Vancouver system of referencing, would appear like this:

> The writer has discussed the question of whether or not all clients should attend group therapy sessions in another paper.[1] Other writers have also discussed this issue, most notably Davis[2] and Anderson.[3,4]

References

1. Brown, D. (1987) Does Group Work Make a Difference? *Nursing Times*, **3**(5), 67–8.
2. Davis, L. (1989) *Against Groups*, Pan, London.
3. Anderson, P. (1990) Group Therapy for In Patients. *British Journal of Group Work*, **2**(4), 34–46.
4. Anderson, P. (1991) *Working with Groups*, Heinemann, Oxford.

The advantages of the Vancouver system are that it is easier on the eye when you are reading a paper. All you see is a series of numbers and in printed text, these numbers are usually set as superscript (the number is set in small type-face, above the line). Also, you can easily check the reference at the end of the paper by looking up the number. On the other hand, the Vancouver system does not always refer you to the name of the author. Also, it is very difficult to make adjustments to once you try to add references to a paper that you are writing. Each time you add a reference, you upset the numbering system. The Vancouver system of referencing is quite widely used in journals and books and you should refer to the style manual recommended in the section above for details of its idiosyncratic use.

Whatever type of referencing system you use, you must use it correctly and consistently. A common fault is to **mix** the styles and to quote author, date of publication **and** a number in the text. You should avoid this and learn both systems.

Examples of referencing styles to avoid

In reading other people's essays, it is possible to come across all sorts of 'hybrid' styles of referencing. The following are examples of methods of referencing to **avoid**. In each case, the writer has broken the fairly simple rules stipulated under the Harvard or Vancouver formats.

Example 7.1a

ANDREWS (1993) has written extensively about the use of computers in social work. He has suggested, as has JONES (1994), that all social workers should use portable computers for notetaking and record-keeping.

Example 7.1b

Andrews, J. (1993) has written extensively about the use of computers in social work. He has suggested, as has Jones, P. D. (1994) that all social workers should use portable computers for notetaking and record-keeping.

Example 7.1c

Andrews, Peter (1993) has written extensively about the use of computers in

social work. He has suggested, as has Jones, Philip (1994) that all social workers should use portable computers for notetaking and record-keeping.

Example 7.1d
Andrews 1993 (1) has written extensively about the use of computers in social
work. He has suggested, as has Jones 1994 (2) that all social workers should use
portable computers for notetaking and record-keeping.

Example 7.1e
Andrews, 1993 has written extensively about the use of computers in social
work. He has suggested, as has **Jones, 1994** that all social workers should use
portable computers for notetaking and record-keeping.

DIAGRAMS AND FIGURES

In some health service courses, essays may require diagrams. There are two
things to say about these:

- Only use them if they really do illuminate your text in a way that words
  could not.
- Keep them simple. Avoid complicated drawings of circles and arrows. Some
  readers may assume that you are suggesting that there is some sort of mathe-
  matical or spatial relationship between the various elements of a complicated
  diagram.

Health care literature went through a phase of writers including complicated,
circular diagrams. Perhaps these had been borrowed from the business and
educational literatures that also tended to favour them. As a rule, keep them
simple or leave them out all together.

Tables are sometimes essential. If you are referring to numerical data in a
research report, you are likely to need to show some of the numbers. Again,
keep the tables simple. Avoid too many lines. Prefer horizontal lines to vertical
ones and do not show too many numbers in one table.

LAYOUT

How you present your essay is important. Figure 7.1 illustrates the points that
you should consider when planning your essay manuscript. Features of this
layout include:

- wide margins of about 1 or 1.5 in;
- double spacing;
- indented paragraphs after the first under each heading;
- bold or underlined subheadings.

ASPECTS OF AIDS AND HIV

John Brown: September 1996

The number of people being diagnosed as being HIV positive or having AIDS is increasing. There is growing evidence that HIV is spreading in the UK by various means in both heterosexual and homo-sexual populations (Johnson, 1988; Donoghue et al., 1989, Pye et al., 1989). At the moment, for many nurses, AIDS is a condition that they read about. It is likely, in the future, that many nurses will find them-selves caring for people with AIDS (Pratt, 1988; Hancock, 1991).

Given the unlikelihood of a 'cure' being found for the condition, at least in the short term, it is possible, too, that at a later date, most nurses and health professionals will have personal experience of knowing someone who is HIV or who has AIDS (Connor and Kingman, 1989; Miller, 1990). At present, it seems that AIDS is some-thing that most people have heard of. Fairly quickly, it is becoming something that many people know a little about. The next stage is possibly that each person will know someone with AIDS.

The changing picture

Whilst there are indications that people are beginning to listen to the call for safe sex, there is also evidence that people associate AIDS with being homosexual and that moral positions are still being held (Wellings and Wadsworth, 1990, Fitzpatrick and Milligan, 1990). Whilst the notion of AIDS as punishment meted out by God is less popular now, it is still possible to find those who are ignorant about the condition and less than sympathetic to the people who have it (Gaze, 1987; Frankenberg, 1990). Wellings and Wadsworth (1990) reporting British Social Attitudes noted that 55% of their respon-dents agreed with the statement that 'AIDS sufferers have only themselves to blame'. It has been suggested that media attempts to change people's attitudes towards AIDS have been less than successful (Kitzinger, 1990). It has also been suggested that AIDS has features in common with epidemics in Europe such as the Black Death of the 14th century (Last, 1988). What is less clear is the degree to which such comparisons add to people's attitudes towards AIDS and AIDS related conditions. For, as Connor and Kingman (1989) point out: AIDS is not, in short, a highly contagious disease, so it is not strictly speaking a 'modern plague', equivalent to the Black Death which decimated Europe in the Middle Ages. (Connor and Kingman, 1990: 3)

These differing viewpoints and perspectives indicate how percep-tions of AIDS vary. Given that these opposing viewpoints are offered by experts in the field, it is reasonable to expect that such diversity of perception also exists amongst the general public and amongst nurses.

Figure 7.1 Example of essay layout.

Gillett offers, amongst others, the following pointers about essay presentation:

1. The question should be accurately written out, at the top of the paper. This is important, not just for the assessor, but also so that in years to come you can clearly identify the subject you were writing about!
2. The date of the assignment and course details, with your name or candidate number should be clearly noted, together with the location of your study centre or institution, if appropriate.
3. The organization of the material should be clear, with logical paragraph construction, appropriate use of headings, wide margins for the assessor to write in, etc.
4. Correct spelling and diligent proofreading are important, as well as good use of English – clear, concise and jargon-free. If you know that your spelling is poor, ask a colleague or friend who can spell to help you. It would be unusual for marks to be deducted for spelling errors, but it can be very irritating to the assessor.
5. A clear original or a good photocopy should be presented, i.e. one that does not have grubby looking pages with words disappearing off the edge of the page.
6. Remember to number the pages.
7. Include an approximate word count.
8. *Always, always keep a copy of any work that you hand in.* It has been known for work to be lost *en route* to the assessor. Remember that one essay may be marked by two or three different people and so the potential for it being lost is quite high! (Gillett, 1990: 93)

PLAGIARISM

Avoid plagiarism like the plague: the name, alone, should put you off. Plagiarism is the attempt at passing off someone else's written work as your own. In other words, copying straight out of books, articles and papers. It is not permitted in any sort of written work, although it crops up mostly in essays. To plagiarize is to break copyright, it is illegal and is one of the very few things that can get you thrown straight off a university or college course. Sometimes, it is done unwittingly. Some people take notes directly out of books and papers and then transfer them into essays. Others, I think, don't **know** that it is wrong to copy directly. Nor is plagiarism always clear-cut. In the following examples I show varieties of what is and what is not plagiarism: with a borderline case in between.

Sample text

The following is an (imaginary) piece of text from a book called *Counselling for Health Workers* by Allan Jones, published in 1994 by Jacobs & Jacobs, London.

There are debates about whether or not counselling 'works'. Various outcome studies have been conducted (e.g. Davies, 1992; Andrews, 1993; Jowett, 1993) in which researchers have tested clients both before and after counselling sessions as an attempt to try to establish (or otherwise) the efficacy of counselling. The problem with undertaking these sorts of studies is that they cannot control all of the variables that are present. Do clients get better because of counselling or do they 'just recover'? Do their families help them and support them while they are being counselled? What is it that 'works'? The counselling or the relationship that they have with the counsellor? All of these things (and, no doubt, many others) make outcome studies difficult.

Outright plagiarism

In the following example, a student has simply copied out the above text and included it, without any sort of reference, in his own essay. This is an obvious case of plagiarism and, if spotted by an examiner, would land the student in serious trouble.

Research into counselling is difficult. There are debates about whether or not counselling 'works'. Various outcome studies have been conducted (e.g. Davies, 1992; Andrews, 1993; Jowett, 1993) in which researchers have tested clients both before and after counselling sessions as an attempt to try to establish (or otherwise) the efficacy of counselling. The problem with undertaking these sorts of studies is that they cannot control all of the variables that are present. Do clients get better because of counselling or do they 'just recover'? Do their families help them and support them while they are being counselled? What is it that 'works'? The counselling or the relationship that they have with the counsellor? All of these things (and, no doubt, many others) make outcome studies difficult.

A borderline case

The following example shows that plagiarism is not always black and white. Some people quote direct chunks of other peoples work and offer a reference to the original work. In the following example, though, it is still unclear what the student is claiming as his own work and what he is expecting the reader to attribute to Jones.

Research into counselling is difficult. Jones (1994) points out that there are debates about whether or not counselling 'works'. Various outcome studies have been conducted (e.g. Davies, 1992; Andrews, 1993; Jowett, 1993) in which researchers have tested clients both before and after counselling sessions as an attempt to try to establish (or otherwise) the efficacy of counselling. The problem with undertaking these sorts of studies is that they cannot control all of the variables that are present. This means that attempts at really clarifying whether or not counselling makes a difference are likely to be thwarted.

In this example, the student has skilfully (or unskilfully, depending on your point of view) intermeshed Jones's direct words with his own. Some might argue that the inclusion of a reference to Jones's work renders the above example acceptable. The fact is, though, that the student is still passing off Jones's work as if it were his own.

Not plagiarism

The following two examples show how the student might have tackled the issue by using Jones's work but not attempting to claim the words as the student's own.

Example 7.2a

In this example, the student **paraphrases** what Jones has written and makes it clear when he is referring, directly, to Jones work. The student does not quote directly from the work of Jones.

Attempts at trying to find out whether or not counselling works have been problematic. Jones (1994) points out that outcome studies are likely to be difficult because so many variables are at work. Jones suggests that in outcome studies it is difficult knowing whether or not it is the 'counselling' that works or if other factors, such as the client's relatives or even the <u>relationship</u> between client and counsellor contribute to the client getting better.

Example 7.2b

In this example, the student **quotes** directly from Jones's work but makes it very clear that he is using a direct quote by indenting the paragraph and citing the reference and page number. This is not plagiarism but appropriate quotation from another writer's work.

It is nearly always difficult to find out whether or not counselling makes a difference to clients. Jones (1984) writes clearly and at length on this topic. He argues that:

'Various outcome studies have been conducted (e.g. Davies, 1992; Andrews, 1993; Jowett, 1993) in which researchers have tested clients both before and after counselling sessions as an attempt to try to establish (or otherwise) the efficacy of counselling. The problem with undertaking these sorts of studies is that they cannot control all of the variables that are present.' (Jones, 1994: 24)

It is almost impossible to overstate how important it is to guard against plagiarism. In recent years there have been court cases over students who have had their degrees withdrawn after it has been established that their essays and/or dissertations have been found to contain large chunks of other peoples work. If you have any doubts about whether or not you are plagiarizing as you write, check your work with a colleague or a lecturer.

CHECKING YOUR ESSAY

Before you hand it in, it is essential that you read through and check your essay thoroughly. One of the drawbacks of using a word processor is that it allows you to work **too** quickly and easily, once you have learned the program. It checks your spelling (but does not pick up differences between words such as 'there' and 'their'), it allows you to review your work on the screen, before you print it out. And this is not the best way of doing things. In my experience, it is always wise to print out a 'hard' copy of your essay and to sit down, with a pen, and work through it for spelling, punctuation, style and content. What looked right on the computer screen may not look so good when it is printed out. It may, of course, look much better. Giles and Hedge (1994) offer a useful check-list of points for checking an essay, project or assignment:

1. Have you kept your audience in mind throughout your essay?
2. Have you said what you meant to say? Does your writing convey your intended message?
3. Have you been consistent and followed the conventions of the genre in which you are writing?
4. Have you signalled the organization of your text in the most appropriate way?
5. Have you given your writing to anyone else to read in order to make sure they understand it?
6. Are your arguments logical?
7. Have you 'hedged your bets' when necessary?
8. Have you used enough evaluation? Is your evaluation careful and precise?
9. If you know you have trouble with some grammatical points, have you checked these?
10. Has every sentence got a subject and a verb?
11. Do your verbs agree with your subjects?
12. Do your sentences have agreement of tense, number and person?
13. Have you checked your spelling? If you have used a word-processing spell-checker, have you then checked the spelling yourself?
14. Have you checked your punctuation?

BINDING

Unless you are given specific instructions about a particular form of binding for your essay, it is probably better **not** to bind it at all. Binders of any sort add **weight** to a pile of essays and the examiner has to carry them, send them to the external examiner and have them posted back. All this can turn out to be very heavy and expensive if each essay is separately bound. If you **must** use a binder, use a very simple, transparent one. Don't use ring binders or lever arch files. Nor be tempted to file each page of your essay in a separate, plastic cover within a binder. This makes it almost impossible for the marker to write notes on your essay, directly.

The best approach is probably to have a title page on the front of your essay (see Figure 7.2 for an example) and simply to staple the top, left-hand corner of your essay. This, in the end, makes for much easier 'handling' of your essay and will usually be much appreciated by the person who has to mark it.

Whatever you do, don't cut out an illustration from a magazine and stick it on the title page to illustrate your essay.

If in any doubt about any of these issues, check with the person to whom you will be handing the essay. Remember, though, what counts is the **content** of your essay and not your ability to present it in an unusual and arresting way.

FEEDBACK

Unfortunately, there are few standards when it comes to the marking of essays. Nor is there consistency about how much or how little written feedback any given tutor or lecturer will give you about your essay. Clearly, notes at the bottom of your essay such as 'good' or 'well-written' are of little help. The more conscientious marker will go through your essay and offer you some commentary on it. Sometimes, this will be in the form of numbered annotations running through the work. In other words, the marker puts a '1' or a '2' in the margin or your work and on a separate sheet offers you notes about the '1' and the '2'. In this way, he or she can almost engage in a dialogue with you about your work.

Other markers and other colleges award marks for your work according to a grid of some sort. Here, you will be allocated a certain percentage of marks for a particular aspect of your essay. There may, for example, be marks awarded in a similar format to the following:

Use of research	25%
Use of other literature	25%
Appropriate referencing	15%
Critical debate of the issues	25%
Layout and presentation	10%

University of Blackheath
Department of Occupational Therapy
Msc in Health Care Studies

A review of the literature on the history of occupational therapy

Jane Hammersmith

Submitted on 24th December 1995

2496 words

Figure 7.2 Example of an essay cover page.

Whatever method is used, you need to know exactly where you stand in relation to your work. If you feel that the written comments on your essay are not sufficient to allow you to learn from them, make sure that you make an appointment to see the marker and to **discuss** your work. Remember, too, that in many colleges and universities, the initially marking is **provisional**. Most college work is moderated by an external examiner who always has the last word about marks awarded. Make sure you know whether or not your work has or will be seen and moderated by an external examiner. Some colleges and universities also have a system by which you can be asked to attend a **viva** or oral examination of all or part of your work. This is usually done if your work falls along a borderline: between degree classifications, between 'pass' and 'fail' or between 'pass' and 'distinction'.

CONCLUSION

All of the issues relating to writing that have been discussed so far apply to writing essays. Keep sentences and paragraphs short. Write to express your ideas not to impress. Don't try to be clever but express your ideas clearly. The sociologist, C. Wright Mills summed it up when he wrote:

> To overcome the academic **prose** you have first to overcome the academic **pose** (Wright Mills, 1959).

8

Writing theses and dissertations

Research? Anyone can do that.

Student, to the author

DISSERTATION OR THESIS?

Labels can complicate matters. Just so that we are clear about what we are saying, for the purposes of this chapter, a dissertation is what an undergraduate writes in her final year and what a masters student writes as part of the requirements for her degree. The masters dissertation is usually a research report but it is also possible, in some colleges, to complete a literature-based dissertation. In essence, this is an extended review of the literature, although some colleges also ask for the inclusion of a research proposal as part of the dissertation. A thesis is what a doctoral student hands in as the final report of her research.

Following an oral examination (or viva) the doctoral student is awarded a PhD on the strength of the thesis and her performance at the oral.

In the USA and Canada, the labels are reversed. Masters students do theses and PhD students do dissertations.

An undergraduate dissertation in the UK is usually about 10 000 words in length. A taught masters degree dissertation is usually about 20 000. Master of Philosophy dissertations are usually up to about 60 000 words and a PhD thesis can be up to about 100 000 words. In practice, few examiners really want to read a double-volume, 100 000 word pair of tomes. If possible, it is usually better to write to under the upper limit. Some examiners refuse to mark works that are over the word limit. Others have some sort of penalty system for students who write too much. Why make life more difficult? After discussion with your tutor, it is likely that these maxima are useful ones to work to:

Bachelors dissertation:	8500 words
Taught masters dissertation:	15 000 words
Master of philosophy dissertation:	50 000 words
PhD thesis:	60–70 000 words

As far as is reasonably possible, avoid running to two volumes.

CONTENT

As we have seen, a dissertation or thesis is usually also a research report. As such, the report will strongly echo a research proposal. Most such reports will contain the following chapters.

- Abstract: a short statement of less than 200 words summarizing what your dissertation or thesis is about. Use these words carefully. The abstract is all that many people will read of your work. It will appear in abstracting journals and on research databases if it is submitted for a masters degree or PhD. Write the abstract after you have completed your work.
- Acknowledgements. Record your thanks to your supervisor and to your family. Go easy. I read an acknowledgement, recently, to the family dog. This is taking things a little far.
- Introduction. This is a short chapter which offers an overview of what is to come.
- Chapter 1: Literature review
- Chapter 2: Aims of the study
- Chapter 3: Methodology
- Chapter 4: Analysis
- Chapter 5: Findings
- Chapter 6: Discussion of findings
- Chapter 7: Conclusions
- Chapter 8: Applications and limitations
- References
- Appendices

It is not usual to index your dissertation or thesis although I always think that this would be extremely useful. I hope that it becomes a standard feature as more and more people work with word processors. There is rarely any need to go beyond ten chapters. If you do write more than ten, you are likely to be writing rather superficially. Avoid too many appendices: they can appear to be page-filling and often are. Also avoid a bibliography unless your tutor has asked for one. The difference between a reference list and a bibliography is this. A reference list is a listing of all of the works that you have referred to, directly, in your dissertation or thesis. A bibliography is a separate listing of other books that are related to the topic but which are not referred to in your work. In practice, bibliographies are very easy to compile, especially with the use of CD-ROM and other searching facilities. Bibliographies that are compiled in this way are merely a list of books and articles that the researcher has managed to find on the particular topic. Generally, it is better to stick to a reference list only.

What should go in the appendices? There is often debate in academic departments about what should go in and what should be left out of the appendices of dissertations and theses (or even whether or not there should be appendices at all). Sommer and Sommer offer the following list of things that might be included in the appendices of a technical report:

1. Score sheets, questionnaires, or observation sheets used in the study. An exception would be instruments that are commonly used and widely available. These can be omitted.
2. Detailed tables and charts primarily for reference purposes. Tables and figures necessary for the reader's understanding should be placed in the results section.
3. List of technical terms. For a general audience, technical terms should also be defined as they occur in the text.
4. Other relevant documents not essential to the reader's comprehension of the report. These might include the sign-up sheet for recruiting subjects, interviewer instructions, instructions for coding interview data, the follow-up letter to respondents who did not reply etc. (Sommer and Sommer, 1991).

In the appendices of qualitative studies, it is not unusual to include examples of interview transcripts and examples of the coding of those transcripts.

PLANNING YOUR RESEARCH PROJECT

The first thing you will be asked to do when you begin to plan your research is to write a research proposal. It is worth taking some time over this. It is important to bear in mind that your research must be achievable. Most people tend to overestimate what they can do in the time that they have. This is as true of PhD candidates as it is of undergraduates.

THE RESEARCH PROPOSAL

These are the headings that you can use for a research proposal. Check with your supervisor that they are the ones that she would like you to use.

- **Title** Keep this short and descriptive. Avoid 'journalistic' titles such as *The Baby and the Bathwater? Health Care Cuts in the Provision of Community Care*. Instead, consider a straightforward title that tells the reader precisely what your study is about, e.g. *A Descriptive Study of the Economics of Community Care in a Rural Setting*.

- **Rationale** Why do you want to do this research? How does it fit in with what has gone before? This should be about two paragraphs in length and place your research in context.
- **Aims** Write about three research aims. Only use a hypothesis if you are using an experimental design. Only use an experimental design if you really know what you are doing. Take advice.
- **Sample** How will you select out respondents from a total population? In the social sciences, it is rare to be able to contact a random sample. In a descriptive, qualitative study, numbers are not so important as the quality of the responses. Be clear about the sampling procedures for both qualitative and quantitative methodologies.
- **Method** Here you should describe what it is you are going to do. Are you going to do some interviews? Are you going to use a questionnaire? If so, are you going to devise your own questionnaire or will you use someone else's? How will you check for the validity and reliability of your instrument? All of these details should be included in this section of your proposal.
- **Ethical considerations** Will you have to go before an ethics committee? If so, what preparations have you made? Usually, if you are going to include patients or clients in your sample, you will be required to send you proposal to a local ethics committee. Do make sure that you are clear about your responsibilities in this field.
- **Financial considerations** How will you pay for the various aspects of your research? Do not forget that you may have a large postage bill if you send out questionnaires. You will also have to pay for paper and for binding the final report. Do not assume that your college will pay for these things.
- **A short CV** Write a two-page curriculum vitae in which you describe your own background in terms of education, jobs, publications and so forth. The aim of the CV in this case is to support your proposal and to show that you have the relevant experience to complete the research that you have in mind.
- **Timetable** Write out a plan of action. The 'rule of thirds' is sometimes useful here. One third of your research time should be devoted to searching the literature. Another third will be taken up with data collection and analysis. The final third will see you writing your dissertation or thesis. On the other hand, it is also good practice to write up your work as you go.

Writing a research proposal is an important aspect of writing. Take time preparing it and then spend a little time or money in having it laser-printed. Keep a copy for yourself and submit at least two copies to your supervisor.

SUPERVISION

All research projects for degrees and higher degrees are supervised. The supervisor may be allocated to you or you may choose one. Make sure that you both get on together and that the supervisor has the right background to supervise your work.

You should be able to expect certain things from a supervisor. Here is a checklist of things to ask for:

- clear guidance on how to proceed with a particular part of your study;
- regular feedback on any written work that you hand in;
- help with methodology and analysis;
- guidance on how to write up your project;
- support and interest;
- regular meetings.

For your part, you should be prepared to work for your supervisor. The supervisor will not be doing the research for you. She should be able to expect the following from you:

- regular written reports;
- motivation;
- ability to work independently;
- awareness of how to use the method that you have chosen;
- realistic aims that you negotiate together.

Be prepared to compromise. As with most relationships, there needs to be give and take. It is easy to get carried away in research and think that there is only one way to do things. Your supervisor may have other ideas. Listen to her carefully, particularly if she has direct experience of the methodology you are using. Also, do not **expect** your supervisor to do everything for you. It is your responsibility to read up on methods and analysis. It is also your responsibility to be aware of and familiar with the literature in your particular field. It is unrealistic to expect your supervisor to know all about the literature in the area of your study.

REVIEWING THE LITERATURE

One of the first elements in the research process is a review of the literature. The literature review is used to demonstrate a number of things. It can:

- demonstrate your knowledge of the writing and research in your chosen field;
- put your research into context; it can show how your project will contribute (even if only to a small degree) to the available knowledge in the field;
- help you to understand what other researchers have done;
- alert you to particular methodological problems;
- give you a greater understanding of the research process.

First, become aware of how to use bibliographies and abstracting journals in your library. These books list all the recent publications of work within your particular field of study. Also, get to know how to use the CD-ROM. CD-ROM offers you a very quick entry to huge numbers of bibliographic references. Learn how to trim down the numbers generated by the computer to a more manageable size.

Next, make sure that you record every reference that you think may be of use. If you use CD-ROM you can print out the details or you can download them to disk. Then, make decisions about which journal papers or books you will need to order through your library. Before you put in orders, check that the library does not already stock the papers or books that you need. Inter-library loans cost a lot of money. Many academic libraries carry back issues of journals and books that are not displayed. Ask the librarian to show you the 'stacks'.

As you collect offprints of papers and collect books, begin to make detailed notes. Note, particularly, whether a given paper is of one of these sorts:

- **An opinion piece**   These may be editorials or single pages in weekly magazines or journals. Clearly, they only represent one person's opinion and cannot be held to be as 'weighty' as other sorts of publications. Do not use them on their own to support an argument.
- **A theory paper**   These are logically argued and properly referenced papers that present you with a theoretical position or that review the literature. Every so often an academic or researcher will actually publish a review of the literature. These are particularly useful if you are just starting out in a field of study. They are useful, too, as role models for the writing of your own literature review.
- **Research reports**   These are probably the most useful sorts of paper. They tell you what research has already been done. They tell you about the sample, method and analysis of findings. They present and discuss the findings and also lead you to the literature.

On your reference cards or in your computer database, make notes of which sort of paper you are dealing with. Then, make notes of what is in a particular paper. If you are likely to want to use direct quotations from the paper (and always use these sparingly) make a careful copy of the quotation and write down the page number next to it. Always offer page numbers when you make reference to direct quotations in your report.

Gash (1989) offers particular reasons why you should work more often with journal articles than with books when carrying out a search of the literature. She suggests that the significant characteristics of this type of publication are as follows:

1. Journals contain the most recent material on the subject. This is because journal issues are published far more quickly and frequently than books.
2. Journals are able to publish papers that are too short, too ephemeral, too controversial or too obscure to warrant publication in book form. The commercial success of a journal does not depend on the demand for one paper in one issue. A book must sell on its own merits.

3. Collectively, journal literature will give an overview of the current state of a subject. Retrospectively, it will enable past trends to be identified and followed. (Gash, 1989)

WRITING UP

When you write up your research review, try to avoid the rather dull listing of everything you have read. The aim of a literature review is not only to identify what you have read but for you to offer a **critical review** of what you have read. Therefore, you should become aware of shortcomings of method or analysis in a research report. You should also be aware of faulty argument or logic in theory papers. You should never just list what you have read, as in the extract in Figure 8.1. Instead, comment on the findings that you report. Offer a critique of the sampling, methodology and findings that the researcher offers. Indicate in what ways those researchers findings fit in with your study.

A **critical** review might read something like the passage in Figure 8.2.

Brown (1987) found that 60% of college students under the age of 21 had dental caries. Davis (1989, 1990) also carried out research that supported this finding. White (1987) suggested that college students do not brush their teeth as often as they should, whilst Andrews (1990) reported that most young people do not change their toothbrush frequently.

Figure 8.1 How not to write a literature review.

Brown (1987) in a study of 200 college students in a North American college found that 60% of his sample had dental caries. It is important to note, though, that Brown used a convenience sample and this may have affected the outcome of his study. In other studies, Davies (1989, 1990) replicated Brown's study with much larger and randomly selected samples. While Davies found that large numbers of students had dental caries, he found that, in government surveys, <u>most</u> young people between the ages of 12 and 21 were reported to have at least one carie. Davies noted, too, a far wider range of possible causes for caries in the under 21 year old age group than did Brown. Following Davies's recommendation that researchers should be cautious in drawing conclusions from small scale dental studies, the present researcher is limiting his study to a review of the research literature on dental work between the years 1990 and the present.

Figure 8.2 How a critical review might be written.

If you keep your reference cards or database system up to date, you will be able to sort your references into an order. Thus, you will find that you can organize your literature review under a series of headings and subheadings. Here, for example, is an extract of the **ordering** of literature review about counselling:

1. **Definitions of counselling**
Client-centred counselling
Prescriptive counselling
Other types of counselling

2. **Humanistic psychology**
History
Carl Rogers
Humanistic principles
Objections

3. **Counselling skills**
Client-centered skills
Six category intervention analysis
Questioning
Reflection
Empathy building
Checking for understanding

4. **Counselling and the health professions**
Counselling in medicine
Counselling in nursing
Counselling in occupational therapy
AIDS counselling
Genetic counselling
RELATE (Marriage guidance)

WHAT A LITERATURE REVIEW LOOKS LIKE

Many people, when they start working on writing up a dissertation or thesis, worry about how to start because they are unsure what a literature review 'looks' like. It is often possible to have a look at other people's dissertations or theses in the local college or university library. In the end, though, there is a variety of different styles that can be used. Figure 8.3, by way of an example, offers the beginning of an imaginary literature review on a dissertation that is about group work in the health care professions.

Introduction

In the past twenty years, much has been written about the importance of clear communication in the health care professions (see, for example, Brown, 1978, 1980; Davies, 1980, 1981; Smith, 1985: Walker, 1990). The group format is an economical one in terms of both time and resources (Walker, 1992). In the small group, a number of people can communicate, quickly, with others. The group format can be used for communication in educational settings (Anthony, 1993), therapy contexts (Evelyn, 1983; Arthur, 1992) and as support systems (Brown, 1989; Davies, 1990).

In this first section, the following issues are discussed: the structure of small groups, group facilitation and the process of assessing the value of group work. In the second section, a review of the research into group work is offered along with a critical review of the use of groups in health care settings.

The structure of small groups

For the purposes of discussion, therapy, support and learning, the 'small group' is often described as being composed of fewer than 20 participants (Andrews, 1985; Smithers, 1990; Webb, 1993). As Webb (1993) pointed out, the advantages of such small numbers are clear: each person can have his or her say, issues and problems can be shared, the group can be reasonably easily managed and group members develop a sense of group identity. Others have also argued that there is a range of psychological advantages to encouraging people to communicate and work in groups (see, for example, Hampton, 1992; Anderson and James, 1993, 1994) and these will be discussed in some detail later in this review.

On the other hand, the small group can be problematic. For those who do not 'belong' to the group, the small group can appear claustrophobic (Webster, 1993). While Webster was referring, in particular, to group therapy, his comments were supported by Davis (1992) who, in a study of 240 student occupational therapists, found that the quieter members of the group often wished that they could leave it and join in a more 'anonymous' lecture. Andrews (1989), reviewing a number of studies into group participation, also reported that when one or two members were of a very different age to the majority of group members, they often felt left out. Again, the issues of inclusion and group identity will be discussed, in greater detail, below.

In health care settings, there have been various reports of work in small groups of under 20. Jones (1994) reported that small group work can be useful in helping to support junior doctors working in stressful environments. Andrews (1992) described the use of small groups for helping people with mental health problems in community settings while Jackson (1987) discussed the use of small therapy groups in in-patient, mental health settings. Jenks and Henderson (1993) argued for more research into the effectiveness of such groups and it is notable that what all the preceding papers have in common is that they were case studies of group work. None of them referred, directly, to research into groups or group work.

Figure 8.3 Example of part of a literature review.

This is, of course, not the only way to write up the literature. As you read it through, you may have your own thoughts about the style and the use of references. Some might question the use of the 'overview' in the introduction or even the use of subheadings. However you do it, you have to find a way of 'laying out' what has been done before: both in the literature and through research. Also, that review should not merely be a 'list' of what has already been written, it should also offer critical commentary.

There is probably no such thing as the **ideal** literature review. While the better ones will be exhaustive in their coverage of what has gone before, no two are likely to be the same. If they were, we could simply record 'standard' reviews of various topics onto floppy disks, give away the copyright on them and encourage students to load the 'standard' review into the front of their dissertations or theses. The point of a literature review is also to illustrate how the student has thought about a particular field, how he or she does or does not understand the context of his or her study and to demonstrate the ability to summarize previous literature.

All of the issues discussed in previous chapters about how to write apply to the writing of a literature review. Remember:

- write short sentences;
- write short paragraphs;
- use simple words;
- define what you mean, as you go;
- be critical of what you read and write;
- aim to communicate and not to impress.

Again, all of the things that apply to writing a literature review, apply to writing the other chapters of your research report. If you use the layout in Figure 8.3 for your report, you are likely to find that it is quite easy to head towards the word limit imposed on you. You will have to be selective about what you include and what you leave out.

At all times, bear in mind that your research report should not only convey your findings but should layout your methodology so clearly that another researcher could work through your report and repeat the process that you worked through. It should be that clear. Also, you should at all times be aware of the weakness of your study. For examples of clear, easy-to-read and easy-to-replicate (at least in theory) studies, look at some of the psychological studies that were carried out 20 or 30 years ago. Consider, for example, Sidney Jourard's (1971) reports of his studies into self-disclosure. Recently, a colleague and I replicated some of Jourard's work and found it quite easy to work through his writing and replicate what he did almost exactly (Burnard and Morrison, 1992). You should aim at this sort of clarity.

A PARTICULAR USE OF FOOTNOTES

In previous chapters, I have suggested that, as a rule, it is not a good idea to use footnotes. They are distracting to the reader and have generally fallen into disuse. However, there are times, in the reporting of a **qualitative** study that they can be useful. Qualitative methods have been widely described in the literature (see, for example Glaser and Strauss, 1967; Field and Morse, 1985; Bryman, 1988; Burnard and Morrison, 1994). It has been suggested that qualitative methods describe what **sorts** of things there are in the world, while quantitative methods describe **how many**. Qualitative research reports individual's perceptions, their subjective experiences and opinions.

Footnotes can be useful as a means of offering **commentary** on a piece of transcript of an interview. Most top-level word-processing programs can easily generate footnotes and will take care of their management. If, for instance, you remove a particular footnote, the rest will automatically be renumbered.

Commentary can be at the level of a discussion of certain aspects of the interview or it can involve an elaboration of what has been said by a particular respondent in the study. Such annotated interview transcripts can be used, in an appendix in the dissertation or thesis, to illustrate an example of one interview. Alternatively, such transcripts can be used as part of the **reporting of findings**, in the main body of the text. Figure 8.4 offers an example of the use of footnotes in annotating a research transcript.

Researcher: Could you tell me a little about the training that you had as a counsellor?

Respondent: I trained for three years as a client-centred counsellor[1] – that was about five years ago. Then I did a short gestalt therapy[2] course. I suppose that I mostly use a humanistic approach[3] that is basically client-centred. I don't believe in the psychoanalytical approach.[4] I'm not sure that it's necessarily a good thing to always harp on the past like that. I know it suits some people but I ... anyway, I would have to have further training in that sort of thing if I was to use that approach.[5]

Researcher: What do you <u>do</u> as a counsellor?

Respondent: That's a big question! Well, I do lots of things. I mean, first and foremost, I <u>listen</u>[6] to the client.[7] I think that listening is all important, really. You can <u>say</u> all sorts of things but the impor-

tant thing is that the client feels lis-
tened to. What else? Well, I use 'reflection'[8] a lot. I sort of echo back to the
client what he or she has said. I think
it can sound a bit daft if it's not used
well. You know – the client is likely to
say 'that's what I just said!' if you
use it too much. In the end, though, I
think it helps to keep the client 'on
track'. It helps them to continue talking about a particular thing. That's
important if you want to go deeper ...

Researcher: What does it mean to 'go deeper?'

1. An approach to counselling developed by Carl Rogers (1952, 1967,
1983). He first called it 'non-directive' counselling and later
'client-centred'. Generally, the aim is not to offer advice or to
'interpret' what the other person says but to help the other person
to make his or her own life-decisions.

2. Gestalt therapy, a particular type of humanistic therapy developed by Fritz Perls. Sometimes described as an existential philosophy. It puts considerable emphasis on the 'client' making his or
her own decisions based on developing self-awareness through noticing small and large physiological, psychological and perceptual
changes.

3. 'Humanistic psychology', often described as the 'third force' in
psychology, to distinguish it from psychodynamic psychology and
behavioural psychology. It focuses, particularly, on subjective,
human experience. Carl Rogers, founder of the client-centred
approach to counselling, was a key figure in the humanistic
psychology movement. The movement is thought to have been named by
Abraham Maslow, American psychologist, probably best known for his
'hierarchy of needs'.

4. The psychoanalytical approach: part of a wider, psychological
approach known as the psychodynamic school of psychology. The term
'analytical' usually refers to that of Jung. The various approaches
usually moot the existence of an 'unconscious' mind that is not,
readily, accessible to the individual, but which may be accessed
through various forms of therapy - most notably through psychoanalysis itself. It is notable that the respondent 'does not
believe in it'.

5. Training as a psychoanalytical therapist usually involves entering a 'training analysis' - the therapist must first be analysed.
It is questionable whether or not the respondent would remain a
counsellor if she undertook this training. It seems more likely
that she would then be operating as a therapist. This raises interesting questions about the differences between counselling and
psychotherapy - issues taken up later in the interview. For a
critique of both client-centred and psychodynamic therapies, see
Masson (1989) who argued that all therapies involve the imposition
of the therapist's values on the client.

6. The idea of listening being a central feature of counselling is

emphasised in much of the counselling literature (see, for example, Rogers, 1967; Heron, 1983; Burnard, 1990).

7. Note the use of the term <u>client</u> to describe the person who receives counselling. The term was probably first used by Carl Rogers in place of the term <u>patient</u>. It is widely used in counselling circles and, to a lesser degree, in psychotherapy.

8. A device, technique or skill widely used in counselling. It involves repeating back the last few words that the other person has spoken to 'jog' them to say more. Also widely used in television interviews. The respondent alludes to how 'artificial' it can seem if overused.

Figure 8.4 Use of footnotes in the annotation of an interview transcript.

STYLE OF A RESEARCH REPORT

Writing a dissertation or a thesis is different to writing a book, article or paper. Polit and Hungler (1991) offer useful advice about the **style** of a research report:

> A scientific report is not an essay but rather a factual account of how and why a problem was studied and what results were obtained. The report should generally not include overtly subjective statements, emotionally laden statements, or exaggerations. When opinions are stated, they should be clearly identified as such, with proper attribution if the opinion was expressed by another writer. In keeping with the goal of objective reporting, personal pronouns such as 'I' and 'my' and 'we' are often avoided, because the passive voice and impersonal pronouns do a better job of conveying impartiality. However, some journals are beginning to break with this tradition and are encouraging a greater balance between active and passive voice and first person and third person narration. If a direct presentation can be made without sacrificing objectivity, a more readable and lively report usually will result. (Polit and Hungler, 1991)

It was noted, earlier, that the rule against the 'first person' in journals is, quite quickly, being revised. It is also not uncommon for qualitative research reports to be written – at least in part – in the first person, with the researcher reporting his or her findings directly.

EVALUATION

What makes a good dissertation or thesis? The point has been debated frequently in universities and colleges and in the literature. Hansen and Waterman (1966) and Howard and Sharp (1983) offer the following criteria for judging your own and other's research:

1. Evidence of an original investigation or the testing of ideas.
2. Competence in independent work or experimentation.
3. An understanding of appropriate techniques.
4. Ability to make critical use of published work and source materials.

5. Appreciation of the relationship of the special theme to the wider field of knowledge.
6. Worthy, in part, of publication.
7. Originality as shown by the topic researched or the methodology employed.
8. Distinct contribution to knowledge.

Not all of these criteria will need to be applied to all dissertations and theses. There should, for example, be a considerable difference between an undergraduate, final-year dissertation and a PhD thesis. The point, of course, is that there are no laid-down guidelines for exactly what this difference should be. Most people, when asked about this question (and I have asked a lot of people about it) talk about issues such as 'depth' and 'detail'. In my experience, few academics or others can state clearly what the differences are between different levels of research. This being the case, work through the above criteria and apply them to your own research.

CHAPTER THREE
STAGE ONE: QUALITATIVE STUDY OF PERCEPTIONS

This chapter describes the first part of the data collection and analyses. It explores the following issues:

- The sample,
- Ethical issues,
- Access to the sample,
- The interview method,
- Methods of analyses of the interviews.

Introduction

The chapter describes the first stage of the study in which interviews were carried out to explore a small group of nurse tutors' and student nurses' perceptions of experiential learning.

Sample

It was decided to interview a group of 12 nurse tutors regarding their views of experiential learning. The criterion for inclusion in this group was that the nurse educator claimed to be using experiential learning methods in his/her work with student nurses. Following Bogdan and Taylor's (1982) suggestion about obtaining respondents, the researcher often asked the person who was being interviewed to recommend another person whom that respondent knew to be using experiential learning methods. This has also been called the snowballing approach to selecting a sample (Field and Morse, 1985).

The snowballing approach was felt to be the best way to gain access to respondents who might talk authoritatively on the topic in hand. It was in line with the researcher's intention to explore the perceptions of people who were using or subject to experiential learning methods.

Figure 8.5 Example of a dissertation layout.

LAYOUT

As with essays, books and anything else you write, how you layout your thesis or dissertation is important. Figure 8.5 illustrates the usual format for layout.

Note the following features:

- wide margins;
- double spacing;
- clear subheadings;
- indented paragraphs after the first under each heading or subheading or 'double-double' spacing between paragraphs.

PUBLISHING

The final stage of the research process is the publication of the findings. This is an important element of research: the publication makes your findings available to other researchers just as you depended on others when you began your litera-ture search. There are a number of ways of publishing your findings. Here are some of them:

- **As a 'short report'**   A number of journals publish a brief report of recently completed research. Sometimes there is payment for such reports. This is unlikely to be the case in the heavyweight journals.
- **As a journal paper**   Here, you submit your work to an academic journal. As we noted in another chapter, it is usual practice for such journals to have submissions reviewed 'blind'. That is to say that the editor sends your manu-script to two other reviews, without disclosing your name. She then takes guidance from them as to whether or not your work should be published. You may be asked to rewrite part or all of your paper before it is published. If asked, do so.
- **As a series of papers**   In this case, you publish your methodology, your findings and various discussion papers as separate entities.
- **As a monograph**   There are a number of imprints of larger publishing houses (e.g. Avebury) who print hard-backed monographs from camera-ready copy supplied by the researcher. Such companies may not offer you royalties but will guarantee speedy publication of your work. Again, such imprints usually seek advice on the quality of your work.
- **As a standard, commercial book**   In this case, you are likely to be asked to rewrite some or all of your research report to make it publishable. Be prepared to do this and read the chapter on writing books. Few, if any, publishers, are likely to publish an entire dissertation or thesis, with the exception of the monograph series described above.

Do get your work published. You will enjoy seeing your work in print and so will other people. You are adding to the body of knowledge only if other people have access to your work. Also, having publications on your CV will make a difference to your career prospects, particularly if you intend teaching in a college or university or if you want to do more research.

Writing articles

9

I don't want to take up literature in a money-making spirit, or be very anxious about making large profits, but selling it at a loss is another thing altogether, and an amusement I cannot well afford.

Lewis Carroll to his publisher

No man but a blockhead ever wrote, except for money.

Samuel Johnson

It has been said before but the best way to learn about something is to write about it. Once you have finished formal courses of teaching and learning, there is often a bit of a gap. There is a tendency to feel that you are in danger of becoming a vegetable. And, of course, you might. One way to lessen the danger is to continue to read and write. Remember the golden rules in the first chapter: read, read, read, write, write, write. Here are some reasons why a health professional might write articles:

- to publish a very good essay;
- to express a point of view;
- to share research findings;
- to describe an innovative project;
- to see your name in print;
- to continue to enjoy the process of writing;
- to earn some money.

Writing articles differs from writing essays. In this chapter we explore some of the technical details involved and examine the process of submitting work for publication.

WHERE TO PUBLISH

Where you hope to publish your work depends on what sorts of articles you intend to write. The following are examples of outlets for your work:

- weekly magazines related to your field of the health professions;
- learned journals associated with your discipline;
- small 'fillers' for magazines;
- a regular column in a weekly magazine.

The last two come in that order as you are not likely to break into the fillers and regular column market until you have a considerable record of publishing in one or both of the first two. Writing articles for weekly magazines is different from writing papers for learned journals and the process of having your article dealt with by the publisher is different. Writing in the 1930s, Brande suggested the following:

> Have periodical debauches of book-buying and magazine-buying, and try to formulate to yourself the editor's possible requirements from the type of periodical he issues. (Brande, 1934)

WRITING FOR MAGAZINES

Most sections of the health professions have their own weekly or monthly magazines. In the nursing profession, for example, there are two weekly publications: the *Nursing Times* and the *Nursing Standard*.

Weekly publications are usually looking for articles of 800–2000 words in length. The sorts of articles that are published vary but examples of them are as follows:

- short research reports;
- examples of good practice;
- historical articles;
- short, controversial pieces;
- case studies;
- discussions of current theory and practice debates.

The magazine that you have in mind may not accept articles 'on spec'. Some may only use in-house writers or commission articles from specialist writers. Some publish invitations to writers and these are the easiest ones to judge in terms of the likelihood of your being able to write for them. If your magazine **does** publish such an invitation and it offers details of how to submit a manuscript, follow these to the letter. Do not assume that you can send in a manuscript that **roughly** follows them: make sure it is an exact fit. Do not risk rejection on the grounds that your manuscript was badly prepared.

If there is no such invitation, write a short letter to the editor, outlining the article that you have in mind. Keep the outline to one page of A4 and then wait until you have an answer. Some editors take a little while to respond. Do not worry them. If you have had no reply after about four weeks, try phoning the editorial department of the magazine. If you still get no response, write another letter to the editor. Be warned: editors vary in the amount of feedback they give you. Some send a standard, word-processed letter that has your name on it. Others will give you details of why they cannot accept your submission if they turn it down. It is doubtful if many people will receive the sort of rejection slip that was published by a columnist in the *Financial Times*, who claimed it to be a genuine rejection slip from a Chinese economic journal:

> We have read your manuscript with boundless delight. If we were to publish your paper, it would be impossible for us to publish any work of a lower standard. And as it is unthinkable that in the next thousand years we shall see its equal, we are, to our regret, compelled to return your divine composition, and to beg you a thousand times to overlook our short sight and timidity. (Findlater, 1984)

If you are asked to submit a manuscript or you have sent one to the editor, you will again have to wait some time to hear whether or not your work has been accepted. You may be asked to make modifications to the manuscript and the editor will give you detailed instructions as to how you can do this. On the other hand, your work may be edited in-house. There is no guarantee that the final published article will be exactly the same as your original submission. Also, you will be asked to sign away the copyright of your paper. While, with books, the author continues to hold the copyright, with articles, the publisher owns it.

There may be a considerable delay between having your work accepted and seeing it in print. Sometimes the wait is up to one year.

One, alternative way of seeing your name in print, in some weekly magazines is to write short reports of research that you have carried out. These are usually about 250–500 words in length and contain details of your sampling, methodology and findings.

A thing you should never do is to send off a good essay that you have written for a course. Essays and published articles differ in important ways. First, you will have used the word 'essay' in your essay. Second, the style is likely to be rather 'academic'. The magazine article is likely to be in a 'snappier' style and illustrated with short case studies or examples from practice. Don't expect that a member of the editorial staff will rewrite your essay for you.

Some magazines will pay you for your work and you will receive payment after the article has been published. Rates vary from about £25 to £150. Most pay somewhere in between these two extremes. Some pay nothing at all.

About a month before publication, you will receive page proofs to check. Appendix C of this book illustrates the marks that you should use when correcting proofs. It is important to make a very clear statement here about correcting proofs:

PROOFS ARE ONLY FOR CORRECTING – NOT FOR REWRITING

Changes in the text, at this stage, are very expensive. Make sure that all you do is correct typographical errors. Any other changes should have been ironed out before you sent in your manuscript. If you realize that you have made an important mistake and this has got through to page proofs, ring the editorial department of the magazine and talk through the problem with them.

Be careful about drawing illustrations for your article. While most magazines claim that you can send in 'rough drawings' for translation by their own artists, those artists cannot mind-read. You cannot expect them to 'know' what you really meant by lines in a diagram. Most will stick very closely to your original. If you draw an oval when you meant to represent a circle, the artist will draw an oval. It is a good idea to use simple drawing instruments to make sure that a diagram that you send in is as nearly exactly what you would like to see in the magazine as possible. Alternatively, ask the reprographics department of your college or university to draw the illustrations for you.

Once you have had a few articles published, you could ask the magazine if they would like some fillers. These are short pieces of between 200 and 500 words that the editorial staff can use to fill the bottoms of pages when other articles do not fit the page exactly. They give the opportunity to be controversial, to get something off your chest and to practise writing to deadline. You may be asked to write something at short notice and it is worth building up a small library of pieces that you could use in this way.

After a while, you may also be asked to review other people's submission and to comment on whether or not you feel the editor should publish a particular paper. Deal with this sort of request promptly – you are likely to be paid for the work. Also, be careful about what you write. Remember what it was like for **you** to receive criticism about your work. Treat people gently: egos are fragile, especially when they are attached to writing. Many people (and you may be one of them) find writing very difficult. Do not be too ready to write off someone else's work. Do offer constructive comments on any manuscript you receive and do not simply write back with the comment: 'this is OK, suggest you publish'. Make comments about why a piece should or should not be published and remember that the author is likely to be sent what you have written.

WRITING FOR JOURNALS

The other sort of article writing is for academic journals. Some lecturers will want to concentrate almost exclusively on these sorts of publication for academic reputation is often based largely on the number of journal publications a person has. You may not agree with this state of affairs but it seems to be true. Certainly, in terms of CV development, journal articles will always 'score' higher than articles in magazines. This is reasonable for journal articles are usually concerned with one or more of the following:

- research reports;
- detailed searches of the literature;
- well argued, theoretical pieces.

Nearly all academic journals operate a blind refereeing system. That is to say that your submission will be sent to two peers in the field, without their knowing your name. Those referees will be asked to comment on whether or not your paper should be published. If it is not published but not turned down absolutely, you may be asked to rewrite part of the whole of your manuscript. Pay close attention to what you are being asked to do and make the changes quickly. When your manuscript is returned, it may be sent back to the referees for their opinion on your modified work.

There is a basic format for research-based papers. The following represent headings that you may want to follow in laying out your work.

- Abstract or summary
- Introduction
- Short literature review
- Aims of the study
- Methodology
- Findings
- Discussion
- Conclusions, including limitations of the study and implications for further research.
- References

As always, follow the 'Advice to Authors' that is usually printed inside the back page of the journal. Follow it to the letter. If the advice asks you to double space your manuscript, do not use one and a half line spacing. If you are asked to submit three copies, make sure that you do. If you do not, it is quite likely that the editor will merely write to you to make the necessary modifications before even considering your work. You are unlikely to be paid for any contribution you make to an academic journal and you may have to wait up to a year to see your work in print.

As with other sorts of published work, you will be sent page proofs to correct. It is important that you read these only to make corrections and not to make modifications. Changes at this stage are very expensive and you will not be at all popular with the editor or the publisher if you try to make extensive alterations to the text.

One other thing that you should work at in relation to journal papers is to avoid sexist writing. Don't use 'man' when you mean 'person'. Avoid the generic use of 'man' as in 'mankind'. Also, avoid perpetuating professional stereotypes by automatically referring to nurses as she or to managers as he. On the other hand, don't get silly about it. Try to avoid really clumsy constructions such as the famous (and probably apocryphal) 'personhole cover'. Your aim is to communicate and not to offend. Nor is your aim to draw attention to your writing by adopting a purposely odd style.

Spend some time in laying out your work. Avoid footnotes and endnotes wherever possible. Anything that is important enough to go into a footnote can be written into the body of the text. This comment is particularly relevant in these days of word processors. Perhaps when people had to type their work, there was an excuse. To integrate a comment meant to retype the whole page, where a footnote could be added to the bottom of the page. Footnotes have gone out of fashion and few, I suspect, mourn their passing. Unfortunately, many of the larger commercial word-processing packages contain the necessary functions to create footnotes and some writers feel obliged to use them because they are there. Resist the temptation. Your paper will be better for your restraint and the editor will prefer it.

Also, avoid the temptation to pad out your work with high-flown sentence construction. Avoid such clichés as 'there is a sense in which' or 'it may be argued by some commentators that ...' Try to write directly and to the point. Keep your sentences short and also your paragraphs. If you are writing a research report, stick to clear description. As I have indicated elsewhere, a student coming to your journal article should find enough information to set about a replication. Read some of the early psychology and sociology reports as role models for clear writing. You may not agree with their research methods nor the ethics of some of their experiments. Often, though, their writing style is excellent.

Send your manuscript to one journal at a time. If it is rejected by one journal, send it to another. If it rejected by the second, reread it, adapt it and send it to a third. If the third rejects it, ask for candid comments from colleagues about ways in which you could improve or adapt it. Remember that some famous book manuscripts were rejected many many times. So it is, sometimes, with academic journal manuscripts. Keep at it. You may have to: your job may depend on it.

One way to overcome the rejection problem is to co-write papers with people who already have a publication record. This can be a useful educational experience for both parties for writing with another person means compromise. You cannot simply write what you like: you have to take into account what the other party feels. Be aware, though, that some university interview panels, when toting up publications, make a note of how many publications you have managed 'solo' and how many are joint publications. Avoid attaching your name to a long list of other people's. Try to write with one other person or on your own. This does not apply, of course, if you are part of a large research project in which it has been agreed that all of you will share publication authorship. It can all become rather clumsy, though and it may be better to divide the publications between you.

After you have had some journal papers published, you may feel brave enough to tackle a book. Again, you have the option, here, of the following:

- writing the book yourself;
- writing it with one or two other people;
- editing a volume with chapters contributed by a number of people.

In my experience, the last often seems the most attractive but offers the hardest work (unless you really find writing difficult). Editing other people's prose is not easy. You have to be both rigorous and tactful. Such a balance is difficult to achieve and it is usually possible and easy to upset someone in the editing process. Also, with an edited volume, there is often a difference between what people tell you they will write and what they actually write. A worse possibility is that the person who told you they will contribute a chapter changes her mind. It happens, so be ready for it. All of this and more is discussed in the next chapter – about writing books.

10

Writing books and reviews

Zest. Gusto. How rarely one hears these words used. How rarely do we see people living, or for that matter, creating by them. Yet if I were asked to name the most important items in a writer's make-up, the things that shape his material and rush him along the road to where he wants to go, I could only warn him to look to his zest, see to his gusto.

Ray Bradbury

That is what you have to have to write a book: zest and gusto. A book is like an article only longer – considerably longer. All the rules of article writing apply to the writing of non-fiction books. And it is non-fiction that is discussed in this chapter. If you are planning to write a novel then you will have to look elsewhere for information.

Why should you want to write a book if you are a health professional? The reasons may be similar to article writing but there are some additional reasons. A short list might include:

- because there is no book on the market that covers this particular aspect of the profession;
- because the profession needs a new book on the topic;
- because you have done research on which you need to elaborate;
- because you have an idea for a book which you think is a good one;
- because you like writing and want to write a book;
- because you have been approached by an editor;
- because you want to convey some of your own zest and gusto to other people.

There are no doubt numerous other reasons. Try to identify why **you** want to write a book. Also, consider the second to last reason in the list above. You need to **want** to write a book and not simply **like the idea**. While I suggested, a little fatuously, perhaps, that writing a book is a bit like writing an article, the point is that a book is much, much longer. You need to have stamina. As a starter, let's consider what an average non-fiction book comprises. Here is a fairly reasonable standard description:

- between 50 000–100 000 words in length;
- between 10 and 12 chapters.

Put like that, it looks a bit daunting. Let us consider the lower end of the scale (and few editors or publishers will consider a manuscript **less** than 50 000 words in length). Supposing your book has ten chapters. Then each chapter will be about 4500 words in length. The extra words will be taken up by appendixes, bibliographies and an introduction: all the words in the book count. Put like that, it may not seem so bad. Again, the keynote is structure. Nobody that I know sits down and starts, from scratch, at page one. The process of getting an idea for a manuscript also mitigates against such an approach. In the field of non-fiction, you don't write the book first. First, you have to have a contract from a publisher. That means two things. The publisher has to be behind your idea. Then, you have to write a detailed proposal about the sort of book you want to write. You may also be asked to write sample chapters. All this is good news for you. The process of preparing a proposal is the process of structuring a book. In this chapter, I will write in some detail about the planning of a proposal and working through that proposal.

THE PROPOSAL

In essence, a book proposal is a book plan. It tells the editor that you have done some homework. You have surveyed the field, you have considered the opposition and you have a chapter-by-chapter plan of what you intend to write. You need to spend some time working on a proposal. After you have written it, you have to convince a publisher that it is worth her while publishing what you write.

How do you contact publishers? There are a number of routes. Here are a few.

- You ring up a publisher who you know deals in works like the one you have in mind and ask for the name of the commissioning editor. Then you write a letter to that editor asking if she would read your proposal.
- You ring the commissioning editor directly and ask the same question. This is one of the best approaches. Ring the company first, and find out the **name** of the commissioning editor and then ring that person directly. It is usually best to work on a 'personal' basis in these matters.
- You talk to someone who has had a book published and you ask them to introduce you to a commissioning editor. You **may** get taken out for lunch by that editor but this is becoming a rare occurrence. I cannot remember the last time I was taken out for a meal by an editor although some have threatened to.

- You are visited by an editor, at work. This happens quite often in university and college departments. Editors like to visit such places to try to persuade academics and their colleagues to submit proposals for books. I don't know what the success rate of this approach is.
- If you are an expert in your field, an editor may approach you to ask you to write a book.

Be prepared for a polite refusal and don't nag. The commissioning editor knows the field and knows what does and does not sell. If she really is interested, she will not risk letting your proposal get away. If you are turned down first time, contact three or four other editors before you reconsider what might be wrong with your proposal. If possible, have someone who writes look through your plan with a critical eye. Then, accept what they say and rewrite it. You have to be prepared to eat bowlfuls of humble pie in the book business. For that is what it is: a business. You will often be asked to rewrite. You will often find that your work is edited with a heavy hand. Accept this. If you don't you will not get published. If you write a huge best-seller, then you might be able to ignore this advice. In the meantime, this is a case of doing as you are told. Publishers invest thousands of pounds in your proposal, if they accept it. It is they who call the shots. Mostly, too, they are right. They know what sells and what sits on shelves. You don't want your book to do the latter. Never believe people who say, 'I just want to get a book published.' What they mean as soon as they have had a proposal accepted is 'I want to write a book that sells.'

Just to recap, before identifying how to write a proposal. First, make sure that you really do want to write a book and are not just in love with the idea. Second, contact a publisher and get agreement to have your proposal read. Three, accept the comments that the publisher makes, if they are interested in your proposal: if not, send it off to another. Four, read any comments that the editor makes and incorporate them into a revamped proposal. It is important not to give up. If your idea for a book is good enough, it **will** be accepted for publication. Also, the better your initial proposal – and the more detailed – the easier it will be to write. For the structure and detail of the proposal will give you a useful framework around which to base your book.

WRITING A PROPOSAL

Most publishers mean the same sort of thing when they ask you for a proposal. They want a short document that identifies the following things:

- the name of the proposed book;
- the author;

- a rationale for the book;
- the market;
- details about the author;
- comparison with other books in the field;
- contents;
- details of length, date of submission and so on.

Wells (1981) offers a useful checklist of things to think about when preparing a book proposal. He suggests, among other things the following points:

1. Have you clearly identified the target reader?
2. Have you explained why the reader needs your book and how he will benefit from it?
3. Have you explained why you are well qualified to write the book?
4. Have you described your proposed book in the best possible terms?
5. Have you covered the whole of the subject, or should you reduce the stated scope to match the coverage?
6. Have you made clear that the book will meet all the requirements of the appropriate and specified examination syllabuses?
7. Have you mentioned competitive books – and explained why yours will be better, or at least a valuable alternative?

Wells's book, *The Successful Author's Handbook*, is an excellent guide to all aspects of writing non-fiction books and will be useful to anyone who is preparing to write one – for the first time or the 21st time.

I have decided that the best illustration of a book proposal would be the one I wrote for the first edition of this book (Figure 10.1). It will, I hope, highlight better than detailed paragraphs, the way a proposal looks when it is written. After you have read it through, I will share with you the editor's comments.

Was it accepted for publication without a struggle? Well, yes and no. First, it was reasonably suggested that in a book of about 50 000 words, 16 chapters were far too many. I was asked, fairly quickly, to resubmit a new proposal in which I cut down the chapters to a more normal ten. Otherwise, the proposal was accepted by the publisher. Incidentally, I sent back a new proposal by return of post. It is important to answer all queries and questions from publishers as quickly as possible. Publishers, like all businesses, work on a tight time schedule. If you want to see your book in print, don't keep them waiting. I don't want to sound like a 'yes' man on these issues but I have found it important and useful to work **with** publishers rather than arguing with them. As I have already suggested, they have published a few more books than you or I are likely to write. They are the experts in the book trade even if you are the expert in your particular field.

Book Proposal: Therapy in Practice Series

Chapman & Hall

Writing for Health Professionals

Philip Burnard, PhD,
Director of Postgraduate Nursing Studies,
University of Wales College of Medicine, Cardiff

Rationale

Health professionals must write. Most need to continually up-date their education and training. Such courses call for essays, projects and dissertations. Health professionals working in colleges and university departments also need to publish. This book would offer a clear and direct guide to all types of writing: from essays to complete books. It would also deal with the ●uestion of using a computer to write – a topic that has been missing from many of the 'how to write' books.

Aims

- To provide a clear guide to all aspects of writing in the health professions.
- To encourage health professionals to write.
  The book would be written in an easy-to-read style with full use made of bullet lists and checklists. Reference would be made to the relevant literature and a full bibliography offered at the end of the book. The overall aim would be a practical one: to help to get the health professional writing. The style would be in keeping with other books in the <u>Therapy in Practice</u> series.

Market

Students and trained staff in all of the health and allied professions, including medicine, nursing, occupational therapy, physiotherapy and others. Educators, tutors and trainers in the health professions. Clinical and community-based practitioners.

The author

Director of postgraduate nursing studies, University of Wales College of Medicine, Cardiff and honorary lecturer in nursing, Hogeschool Midden Nederland, Utrecht, Netherlands. Author of 15 textbooks on communication, interpersonal skills training, coun-selling, research methods, ethics and education. Three titles published in the <u>Therapy in Practice</u> series and another in print. More that 130 published papers and articles in UK and USA. Manuscript and proposal reviewer for three British publishers, five health care journals and book reviewer for four health care journals. Masters degree in education and PhD in experiential learning.

Comparison with other titles

There are a number of general 'how to write' books on the market but these are mostly aimed at specific writing markets: the prospective author or the feature writer. The proposed book would be written especially for the health care worker and would address a wider range of writing projects. The likely competitor in this field would be:
Turk, C. and Kirkman, J. (1989) <u>Effective Writing: Improving Scientific, Technical and Business Communication</u>, 2nd edn, E. and F. N. Spon, London. This is a well written and clear book about how to improve report and business writing. It addresses a different market to the new book.

The book
Words: 50,000
Line diagrams (word illustrations): c. 10
Other illustrations: none
Delivery of manuscript: 6 months from signing of contract or earlier

Contents

Introduction

- Who writes?
- Why write?
- What is in this book?
- How to use the book
- Writing and you

1.Writing: the basics

- Writing in the Health Professions
- Types of writing

- Getting ideas
- Keeping a journal
- Reading
- Rules of good writing
- Writing to order
- Simplicity and structure
- Counting words

2. Equipment and environment

- Basic equipment
- Basic books
- Journals
- Using the library
- The writing environment
- Writing on the move
- Writing and work

3. Buying a computer

- Why use a computer?
- What sort of computer?
- Desktop, laptop and notebook
- Choosing a printer
- Where to buy?
- Writer's software

4. Shareware

- What is shareware?
- A review of shareware programs for writers

5. Writing with a computer

- Choosing a word processor
- Basic structure
- Writing and editing
- Tips on word-processing

6. Keeping databases

- What is a database?
- Database programs
- Fixed field databases
- Free form databases
- Keeping references on computer

- Keeping notes on computer
- Databases and research

7.Educational writing
- Writing and the tutor/trainer
- Preparing handouts
- Preparing visual aids
- Preparing book lists
- Preparing course handbooks

8.Writing essays
- Basic structure
- Brainstorming
- Outlining
- Outlining computer programs
- Research
- Using references
- Writing the essay
- Checking

9.Writing dissertations and theses
- What is a dissertation or thesis?
- Planning your work
- Supervision
- Doing your research project
- Writing up
- Layout
- The finished product

10.Writing articles
- Why write articles?
- The health professional journals
- Instructions to authors
- House style
- Planning your article
- Referencing style
- Writing the article
- Submission
- The refereeing process
- Professionalism
- Journalism

11.Writing books

- Why write books?
- Books and the health professions
- What sort of book?
- Writing a proposal
- Choosing a publisher
- Following a plan
- The writing process
- Indexing

12.Working with publishers

- Editors and journals
- Book publishers and editors
- What happens when you write a book
- Relationship with editors
- Checking proofs

13.Layout

- The page
- The font
- The layout
- Headings and subheadings
- Consistency
- Keeping it simple
- Tables and figures
- Printing

14.Editing

- The writing habit
- Common errors and how to avoid them
- Working through your manuscript
- Cutting and rewriting
- On taking advice

15.Putting it all together

- Reading and writing
- Developing a style
- Doing research
- Structure and simplicity
- Write now!

```
16.Exercises for the writer
```

```
Ten exercises for practising the skills described in
the book, including:
```

- Free writing
- Planning a journal
- Editing a piece of writing
- Planning an article
- Reviewing your writing history
- Writing a book proposal
- Identifying computing needs
- Checking layout
- Criticizing your own work
- Planning for the future

```
References
Bibliography
Index
```

```
September 1991
```

```
Dr Philip Burnard
```

Figure 10.1 Example of a book proposal.

Some publishers ask you to complete a publishing proposal **form** rather than submit your own proposal – although no publisher is likely to reject, automatically, a well-written proposal laid out by a potential author. Such proposal forms usually ask the following questions and clearly, they don't expect 'yes' or 'no' answers to the questions. If you can, have your answers typed into the form, although, oddly enough, this is becoming more difficult in the age of word processors. It is often difficult to 'line up' your word processor with sufficient accuracy to complete forms. I still keep a portable typewriter for filling in forms. The questions that the publisher's proposal form ask are likely to be variants of these:

- your name and qualifications;
- your address and telephone number;
- present appointment;
- precis of career to date;
- previous publications;
- provisional title of the book;
- details of the subject of the proposed book;
- a brief statement about the purpose of the book;

- why the book is needed;
- principle UK market for the book;
- other markets (USA, Europe, etc.);
- for which courses the book would be a required text;
- for which courses the book would be one of a number of required texts;
- for which courses the book would be supplementary reading;
- details of other professional staff who are likely to be interested in the book;
- competitive titles;
- advantages of your book over the above;
- how quickly might the book become out of date?
- approximate number of words required for the book;
- approximate number of illustrations required;
- time required to deliver final manuscript;
- names and address of people would be qualified to give an opinion of your work;
- any further information which might be useful.

What happens to a proposal when you send it to a commissioning editor? First, she reads it through and sees whether or not it would fit into the publishing house's plan and whether or not it is publishable and saleable. Then, if these criteria are satisfied, the proposal is sent to one or more reviewers who are usually experts in the field for their opinions. Like the editor, they may recommend small or substantial changes to the proposal or may suggest its being rejected all together. In my experience, reviewers vary considerably in what they look for and what they write about proposals. Some publishers send the reviewers a standard assessment form. Some just ask for comments. Whatever the case, you will again have to bite your tongue and do what you are told. If you do not, it is likely that your book will not be published. That is not to say that you should become a publisher's doormat but merely to remind you that book publishing is a commercial venture. The publishers are not there to be astounded by your ideas and prose but to sell books.

You may or may not be sent the reviewer's comments to read. If you are, be prepared for something of a shock. Reading other people's comments about your work can be difficult. Most of us, I suspect, are fairly thin-skinned when it comes to criticism, and criticism of **written** work – for reasons I do not understand – can be particularly painful. Not all reviewers bear in mind that the potential author might read their comments – although experienced ones will. Not all reviewers pull their punches when it comes to describing how they feel about particular proposals. I still get an odd feeling in the pit of my stomach when I open an envelope that I know contains a set of reviewers' comments about a proposal (or a completed manuscript). Don't get **too** concerned about it but be prepared.

If everyone is happy with your proposal, you will be sent a contract to write the book. DO NOT BEGIN WRITING UNTIL YOU HAVE SIGNED THE CONTRACT. This is important. The contract is your agreement with the publisher to write a particular book. It may not be the book that you started writing a year ago. Also, you may not get a contract at all. If this happens, it is unlikely that another publisher will be interested in a half-written or completely written manuscript.

THE CONTRACT

The contract that you sign with the publisher is an agreement, on your part, to write a particular book and on their part to publish it within a reasonable time limit. The clauses of a book contract are usually these.

- **The work**   Your manuscript, for the purposes of the contract, will be known rather quaintly as 'the work'. In this clause, the agreed title will be used. The title is not binding and you or the editor may agree to use another one at a later date. Incidentally, titles are not copyright. In theory, you are free to write books called *Gone With the Wind* or *Alice in Wonderland*, though I don't recommend it.
- **Rights granted**   This is a statement that the publisher will have sole and exclusive right and licence to produce and publish your work. The copyright remains yours.
- **Delivery of the work**   This is a time limit for the delivery of the completed manuscript.
- **State of the typescript**   This spells out that you have both agreed a format for the typescript.
- **Illustrations**   This identifies yours and the publishers responsibility for supplying illustrations for your work.
- **Permissions**   This refers to your responsibility for obtaining permission to quote directly from other people's published work. Normally, under the 'fair dealing' agreement, you are able to quote short phrases or sentences from other people's work without written permission. If in doubt, contact the editor.
- **Editing the typescript**   This clause conveys the publisher's right to edit your work into a house style acceptable to both parties.
- **Publishers undertaking**   This is a formal statement that, everything else being equal, the company will publish your book.
- **Author's warranty**   This is the clause that says that the publisher will defend your copyright.
- **Warnings in the text**   This clause acknowledges that if you are going to recommend dangerous exercises or activities that you will publish a warning with them.
- **Liability for author's property**   This clause is a let-out clause for the publisher. It states that they are not insured against their losing of your work. Make sure you keep copies and ask for an acknowledgement of receipt of your manuscript.

- **Competing works**   Reasonably, you are asked not to write a competing book during the time of your agreement with the company.
- **Moral rights of author** This asserts that the work is yours, will be published under your name and that you can object to the way in which your work has been treated by the publisher.
- **Royalties**   This clause spells out what, if any, royalties you will be paid. 10% of the cover price is a usual figure, per copy.
- **Subsidiary rights**   This clause is about the publisher's rights to sell your work to other companies or to sell the film rights. This clause is unlikely to affect your non-fiction book.
- **Accounts**   Here, the publisher tells you how often the company will pay you royalties. At the moment, some companies pay twice yearly, others yearly. The trend is towards once a year payment.
- **Examination of accounts**   Here, you are told that you can examine the companies accounts as they relate to your work. I have yet to meet anyone who has challenged a publisher on this issue but bear in mind that all publishers send you a thorough breakdown of your sales every time they send you a royalties cheque.
- **Presentation copies** This clause tells you how many free copies you will be given when the book is published and at what discount you can buy further copies. Go easy with your free copies when you receive them. I once worked with a publisher that gave me 25 free copies (3–6 is normal) and I handed them out to all and sundry thinking the supply would last for ever. I was down to two copies within a fortnight. In the excitement of receiving your free copies, it is easy to get carried away. It is a good idea to hold back at least **three** copies for your own use. One for your bookshelf. One to show or lend to your friends (and which can be allowed to get dog-eared) and a third copy as a 'spare'. The third copy might be useful as a present for someone, later on, when all the fuss has died down. Don't forget, too, that every book you give away means the potential loss of a **sale**. If you **give** someone your book, they do not have to **buy** it.
- **New editions**   This is about your being asked to produce a second and subsequent editions if the book sells well. Normally, you will only be asked to prepare a second edition after the first has sold well for about five years. Don't confuse **printings** with **editions**. Your book, if it sells well, may be reprinted, as it stands. After five years, you may be asked to update and/or partially rewrite your book. This will be the second edition.
- **Termination**   This outlines the limits to your relationship with the publisher and the grounds for cancelling the agreement.
- **Notice**   This tells you how to terminate the agreement.
- **Arbitration**   This is an important clause. It points out that the agreement is binding under English law and explains how any dispute may be arbitrated.
- **Advance**   This clause tells you how much money the company will pay you in advance of publication and when.

Read your contract carefully. If you have any doubts about clauses in the contract, contact the publisher for clarification. If you write books regularly and work with a variety of publishers, you may want to consider joining the Society of Authors. You can do this once you have had one full-length book published, for an annual subscription. The Society offers a book contract reading and vetting service and it is a very prompt and thorough one. Mostly, though, contracts are fairly standard, along the lines of the clauses discussed above. One clause that may be in your contract and one that you may want to query is one that says that the publisher will have first refusal on your next book. This is rather limiting if you do not want to write exclusively for one publisher. If you do not want to be bound by it, talk to the editor and then strike out the clause. Your signature of the contract will require a witness. Once you have signed the contract you are bound by it.

ADVANCES

Some publishers will allow you an advance on royalties as an incentive. This can take a number of forms.

- A single amount following the signing of contracts. I have found this amount to vary from £100 to £700. Forget any ideas that you will be offered millions.
- An amount following the signing of contracts and an amount on the delivery of an acceptable manuscript.
- A single amount following the acceptance of a suitable manuscript. Note the words 'an acceptable manuscript'. That means acceptable to the publisher. You may be asked to rewrite sections or chapters before you see your advance.
- An amount on publication of the book.

Some publishers give no advances at all. There is one important thing to remember: an advance is just that. What you are paid prior to publication will have to be paid back from the royalties that you earn once the book is published. Therefore, it is wise not to push for high advances (unless you are really broke). If you do, it may be some time before you see any other earnings from your work.

A few academic imprints give you no royalties at all. They publish research monographs for small markets and you have to submit camera-ready copy of your manuscript. That is to say that the copy you submit is the copy that will appear in the finished book. The publisher undertakes to publish your work quickly and to give you a certain number of free copies. These sorts of books are usually hard bound for sales to libraries and universities. You will not make any money but you will see your work in print in a short space of time. This sort of publishing is useful if you want to pass on your PhD findings to a larger audience. Few other sorts of publishers will publish theses as they stand. Some will ask for a major rewrite that you may not want to do. Others will not be interested at all. This sort of publishing enterprise offers a useful service to academics and researchers who might otherwise have to rely only on journal publications.

One sort of publishing to avoid is **vanity** publishing. This is a form of publishing where you pay for everything. The publisher agrees to help you publish your book but you pay for all aspects of the process from reading the manuscript to having the book printed. Most vanity publishers do little to promote their authors and most bookshops will not stock books from vanity publishers. The net result could be that you are stuck with a garage full of unsaleable books. Don't do it. If you book is worth publishing, a 'real' publisher will publish it.

WRITING THE BOOK

There are various things to say about writing a book. These, like other aspects of writing can be divided into stages:

- completing the outline;
- doing the research;
- doing the writing;
- preparing the manuscript;
- sending it to the publishers;
- waiting;
- dealing with queries, the author's questionnaire and proofreading;
- preparing the index.

COMPLETING THE OUTLINE

First, the proposal must be worked upon. All of the headings and subheadings need to be broken down further into manageable and writable chunks. It is a good idea, at this stage, to allocate words to each section and to try to stick to those word limits.

DOING THE RESEARCH

You are unlikely to have enough knowledge in your head to complete the book in one go. This means, rather like writing essays, you must make many trips to the library for references, books and journal papers. Then, you need to file them away in such a way that you both remember them and can find them quickly. Some people have elaborate filing systems. I tend to work in the middle of a pile of papers and books and can usually find what I want. Information for new books can be gleaned from a number of sources. Here are a few:

- research carried out by the writer;
- other people's research reports;
- public and college libraries;
- journal papers and articles;
- life experience;
- your own experience of the health profession;
- interviews.

DOING THE WRITING

Get into a writing habit. If you can, write every day and do not stop until you have reached the target that you have set yourself. You do not have to write the book straight through. Start with a chapter you feel confident about and write that first. On the other hand, do not leave the most difficult chapter until last. Try to end on a chapter that's easy to write. Keep an eye on three things:

- accuracy;
- consistency of style;
- simplicity.

Again, resist the urge to be longwinded or clever. You may be writing 50 000 words but every one has to count. You cannot pad out a book any more than you can pad out an essay. If you do, it is unlikely that people will read it. Most people can spot 'page-filling' a mile off.

If at all possible, write straight into a word-processing program on a computer. This will allow you all sorts of control over the writing and editing process. Write first, fairly quickly. Then go back and edit what you have written.

COPYRIGHT

There is sometimes confusion in people's minds about the question of copyright. You do not have to register or publish a piece of written work in order for it to be considered copyright. The fact that you have written it at all means that you already own the copyright to the work. Note, though, that when you sell an **article** to a publisher, you are often asked to sign over the copyright of the piece to that publisher. This means, in effect, that the publisher can do what it likes with your piece. It may edit it, significantly and it may sell it on to other publishers without, legally, having to tell you. In practice (we hope) most publishers of journals will tell you that they are selling your work to other publishers. In one case, though, I had the experience of opening an American book – in order to review it – only to find that the book contained a chapter made up of an article I had had published in a British journal some years before. Clearly, the journal had sold the piece on, but without telling me. It is difficult to say how widespread this practice is, but it is to be hoped that it happens fairly rarely.

In the case of book publication, the author usually retains the copyright. If you look at the reverse of the title page of most books, you will see that the author's name stands next to the copyright sign © – an indicator that the author still holds the copyright. Incidentally, there is no need to **use** the copyright sign in documents that you produce for other purposes (e.g. reports, curriculum documents, brochures etc.). As we have seen, the writer of these automatically holds the copyright by virtue of having written the document.

On rare occasions, a publisher may ask an author to sign over copyright to that company. In this case, you may want to consider ver / carefully whether or not this is something you are prepared to do.

Sometimes, you will want to quote other people's work, directly, in your own book. The copyright law is far from specific on the question of how much or how little you can do this but one thing is certain: you **must** acknowledge your sources. You must indicate when a piece of writing has been quoted directly from other people's work. Not to do this constitutes plagiarism and legal action can follow such a breach of copyright. The usual format for indicating direct quotations from other people's work is to indent the paragraph containing the quote and to offer, in brackets, the original author's name and the year of publication (in the text) and the full reference to the work from which the quote was taken (in the reference list at the back of the book or at the end of the chapter).

Barry Turner (1992) offers a useful summary of the general principles of quoting from other people's work as follows:

> The rule is, a writer has the undisputed right to quote another writer for 'purposes of criticism or review', as long as 'sufficient acknowledgement' is given. There are limits of course. It is not the done thing to lift a 'substantial part' of a copyright work without permission. Unfortunately, there is little agreement on what constitutes 'a substantial part'... Common sense suggests basing the assessment on the length and importance of the quotation; the amount quoted in relation to the text as a whole; the extent to which the work competes with the work quoted, and the extent to which the words quoted are saving a writer time and trouble.

> Some years ago, the Society of Authors and The Publisher's Association stated that they would usually regard as 'fair dealing' the use of a single extract of up to 400 words or a series of extracts (of which none exceeds 300 words) to a total of 800 words from a prose work, and extracts to a total of 40 lines from a poem, provided that this did not exceed a quarter of the poem. (Turner, 1992)

Bear in mind that when you **do** quote from other people's work, you must quote **exactly** what is written in the original text – including the original punctuation. If you leave out a small section of the text, you indicate this with three ellipses (...) as indicated in the above quotation. If you want to emphasize something of the original text, you do so by placing the words in italics and at the end of the quotation you add the following, in brackets: *emphasis added*. As we have seen, it is not good practice to use the term *sic* after a quotation to show that you have spotted a grammatical error. If the quotation was **that** bad, it was probably better not to use it at all. Incidentally, if the passage **does** contain a grammatical, typographical or spelling error, you must not 'correct' this. Instead, you still write out the quotation exactly as it appeared in the original publication. Again, though, you may want to consider whether or not you use such a quotation.

Sometimes, a publisher will ask you to obtain 'permission' from the publisher of the original text, for use of the quotation(s). In this case, your publisher may supply you with 'permission forms' and you fill in the form as a request to the second or subsequent publishers to ask permission to quote from their books. Those publishers, if they are happy for you to use the quotation(s) will then stamp the form, thus indicating that permission has been granted. In some cases – particularly when the quotation is a 'literary' or poetic one, there may be a charge for the use of a quotation. Also, of course, permission may **not** be granted, although, in practice, this is rare.

It should be noted that no one holds the copyright to book **titles**. Thus, if you publish a book called *Legal Aspects of Health Care Work*, there is nothing to stop another author writing a book with the same title. In choosing your own title, though, it is probably best to do some homework. It is not, generally, good practice to 'borrow' someone else's title. After all, the buyer may end up purchasing the **other** writer's book and you have lost a sale.

Copyright normally lasts for fifty years from the end of the calendar year in which the author dies. This rule applies to unpublished as well as published work.

PREPARING THE MANUSCRIPT

Once you have written the manuscript, you need to make sure that it is in a fairly standard format before you send it to the publishers. Publishers rarely seem to tell you what they want but experience suggests that there are certain rules of layout for a manuscript submission. They are as follows.

- Print on one side of good-quality A4 paper.
- Double space the lines.
- Leave good margins around the edge of your work (about 1.5 in on all sides).
- Put numbers on all pages and number the manuscript consecutively from the first page to the last. Don't start again at 1 for a new chapter. If you need to

insert a few pages before sending off the manuscript, call the new pages 26b ... 26c etc. If there are a number of extra pages, renumber the entire manuscript. Don't forget that your word processor can automatically number the pages for you. I put the number at the bottom of the page, in the centre. I have read that some publishers prefer page numbers in the top right-hand corner. I have not had any complaints.

- Don't use 'headers' or 'footers'. Your aim is not to produce a manuscript that looks like a book but one on which the subeditor can work. She will not thank you if she has to cross out headers and footers on every page.
- Don't use a wide range of fonts. Stick to a standard 10 or 12 pt font throughout.
- Print diagrams on separate pages and don't integrate them with the text. Put the diagram next to the page to which it refers.
- Don't bind the manuscript at the side. Do not staple it but leave the pages free.
- At the top of each page, print your name and the title of the manuscript. This is just in case anyone drops part of it and then wonders to which pile of papers these particular ones refer.

Figure 10.2 illustrates one page of manuscript from this chapter, as I submitted it to the publisher. It illustrates a number of the issues identified in the above list. Notice, too, the indentations that break up the text into paragraphs. There is never an indent at the beginning of a piece of text, under a subheading. The paragraphs following, however, are indented.

THE PREPARATION OF ILLUSTRATIONS

Illustrations are attractive but they are also expensive. Remember that if you want to use other people's pictures, photographs or diagrams you will have to obtain permission to do so. You are likely, too, to be asked by the publishers to supply those illustrations in a format that will allow the printers to print direct from the material that you supply. This, again, can be an added expense.

Photographs, particularly those containing people, can 'date' very easily. Hairstyles and lengths change more quickly and so do styles in glasses and clothes. Try to avoid, particularly, photographs that do not really illustrate any particular point. These are the sort that bear legends such as 'a group of students enjoying working together' or 'many nurses work in the community' and accompany pictures of groups of people doing nothing in particular. This is an expensive way of filling pages.

Simple line illustrations are possibly the most inexpensive choice if you **have** to have illustrations. They consist, simply, of black and white diagrams of a fairly rudimentary nature. 'Box' diagrams, that draw attention to particular points, also fall into this category. Remember that the diagrams that you send in with your manuscript must be a very accurate representation of what you want to see on the printed page. You cannot assume that the publisher's graphical

SIMPLICITY AND STRUCTURE

These remain the keywords. All the best writing is simple in style. All the best writing (except, perhaps, the 'flow of consciousness' writers like James Joyce and Virginia Woolf – but we are not in their league) is structured. A simple writing style is not always easy to achieve. It can be made easier, though, if you try to avoid 'fillers' such as the following:

- there is a sense in which...
- however...
- it is the writer's view that...
- it is sometimes the case that...
- the writer would like to forward the view that...
- we have to consider this over and against the other view that...

All of these hide the message. Sometimes academics use them to try to hedge their bets. It is as if they are saying to the reader: 'I know there are other points of views and this may not be the right one and that there are a whole range of other things that could be said here but...' In the end, we have to be prepared to stick to what we want to say and say it. It really is as simple as that. Mostly we are not writing philosophy so we don't have to ponder over every nuance of meaning and possibility. Take some risks. Declare what you want to say without the wrapping. But...keep it structured.

50

Figure 10.2 Example of a page of book manuscript.

department can 'guess' what you had in mind. If you send in a diagram of particular proportions, you are likely to find that the proofs that you receive echo those proportions. Remember, too, that changes to line diagram proofs can be very expensive. So keep the diagrams simple and make sure that they are accurate. If you feel unable to draw sufficiently good diagrams yourself, enrol a friend or colleague to work on them. Some colleges and universities have a 'graphics department' that can also help. Chapman & Hall (1995) offer the following directions about line illustrations to their authors:

- The artwork should be drawn (or printed) in uniformly black ink on a flat white or transparent background (preferably not stiff board). Avoid lined paper even if the lines are feint – these can sometimes be difficult to lose in reproduction.
- Indicate the figure number and abbreviated book title and/or author's name on the front side of the illustration, outside the image area, using light blue crayons. Please also clarify the orientation of the illustration.
- Outlines should be firm and not too thick (these will appear too heavy on the final printed page) nor too thin (thin lines can break up after reproduction). Stippling or cross-hatching must not be too fine (reduction may cause the shading to fill in and/or break up). Avoid large areas of solid black.
- The size of the original should be no more than twice the intended size on the final printed page unless the thickness of the line is robust enough to survive reduction beyond 50%. Ideally, your original should be × 1.5 larger than its final size on the book page. Enlargement of your original is to be avoided as any flaws/unsharpnesses become exaggerated.

SENDING IT TO THE PUBLISHERS

When you are quite sure that the manuscript is complete and you have checked the spelling, ensured that all pages are numbered and that you have printed out a clean copy, you are ready to send it off to the publisher. If you have no other instructions, send two copies: the top copy and a photocopy. Also, keep a hard copy for yourself. Don't rely on the copy you have on disk. If the editor rings up and asks about something on page 38, it will be difficult to find that page if all the chapters exist only as computer files.

A medium-sized manuscript is best packed in a padded posting bag, well sealed. Enclose a letter outlining what is in the package and post it off. If the manuscript is too large, send it in the box that the paper was packed in. It is a good idea to enclose a self-addressed card to enable the publishers to acknowledge receipt of the manuscript. I have sent off manuscripts and waited for over two weeks to hear whether or not they were received. When I've phoned the publisher, they've told me that they had received it ten days previously. There is no guarantee that publishers will automatically acknowledge receipt, so make it easy for them.

PRESENTATION OF MANUSCRIPTS ON DISK

More and more publishers are accepting completed manuscripts on disk. This can speed up production of your book and can save production costs. On the other hand, most still ask you, also, to send in 'hard copy' – a printed-out version of your manuscript. You may be invited to respond to editors comments by reference to either the disk version of your manuscript or the printed version.

If you are planning to send in your manuscript on disk, there are certain rules that you must follow. These include the following:

- Use a standard, well-known word processor and tell the publishers which one you have used. This is usually discussed in advance of your sending in your work.
- Create a separate file for each chapter and for other sections of the book such as the introduction, preface, bibliography and so on. Give these files readily recognizable names (e.g. CHAP1.DOC, BIBLIOG.DOC).
- Keep illustrations in separate files and name them clearly.
- Keep files reasonably small (about 100K is the maximum). If your chapters are larger than this, divide them into two and name them appropriately (e.g. CHAP1A.DOC, CHAP1B. DOC).
- Be very consistent in your layout and keep the layout very simple. Use one font throughout, if possible, and indicate headings and subheadings in the same font. Keep headings and subheadings to the left hand margin and do not centre text.
- Don't attempt to design or layout the final product. Keep your files as simple text files as far as is possible.
- Don't include diagrams, lines or boxes in the body of the text.
- Avoid footnotes as far as possible. This is good, general writing practice.
- Don't put in 'hard returns' at the ends of lines. In other words, don't press the 'enter' or 'return' key at the end of each line but allow the text to 'word-wrap'. Hard returns should, however, be used at the ends of paragraphs.
- Use the following codes within your text to indicate chapter headings, headings and subheadings:

  <<Chap Head>>   in front of a chapter heading
  <<A Head>>   in front of major headings, within chapters
  <<B Head>>   in front of the next level of subheadings
  <<C Head>>   in front of sub-subheadings.

- As far as possible, avoid any further levels of headings and subheadings.
- Wherever possible, avoid using underlining. Instead, use italics and use that sparingly. Again, this is good general writing practice. As far as possible, avoid using underlining in any manuscripts. Underlining is 'shorthand' for italics and was used on typewriters before italicization was possible.

Some academic publishers will accept your manuscript on disk as camera-ready copy. If you submit a manuscript in this format, bear in mind your responsibility. The printers will use your disk, directly, in the process of printing out the pages of your book. Any mistakes in the layout or typography of the text will be reproduced in the book itself. This is in contrast to the advice and information given in the previous paragraphs. It should be emphasized that **most** publishers will modify your text on disk quite considerably before your book is printed. If you **do** have to submit camera-ready copy on disk, you must spend a lot of time on making sure that the file on the disk will exactly match the way you want your text to appear on the printed page. If it is at all possible, avoid agreeing to submit text as camera-ready copy in this way. On the other hand, as we have seen the supply of **unformatted** text – as described above – can help speed up the production of your book and keep costs down. This, in turn, will help keep down the cover price of your book and this may well mean that you sell more copies.

WAITING

Then the wait. There is usually a considerable time gap between sending off the completed manuscript and hearing anything from the publisher. The temptation is strong to ring and find out what is happening. Do this if it makes you feel better but be assured that the process of book publishing is a fairly slow one. Also, be warned that people in the publishing field tend to change jobs with alarming frequency. You may not finish your book with the editor you started with.

The first thing you are likely to hear from the publisher is the satisfying sound of your advance or royalties cheque plopping onto the door mat. After that, another long silence.

During this period, the following things are happening at the publishers:

- The editor may read the manuscript to see whether or not it is in line with what was expected.
- She will certainly ask one of the reviewers to read it and to comment on it.
- The editor will send for estimates of printing costs. There is a narrow and small profit margin on non-fiction books.

After these things have happened, the editor may write back to you with suggested modifications or rewrites. Do them and do them quickly. Time is all important now for time, at this stage, is money.

Once a complete and satisfactory manuscript is with the publisher, the next stage is that the manuscript is sent to a sub-editor who laboriously works through the entire manuscript checking on the spelling, style, grammar, sentence construction, references and just about everything else in the book.

Jill Baker, in a useful book about copy editing, suggests the following advice to sub-editors about three levels on which to read and correct manuscripts:

1. Word by word, for consistency and conformity to style, correct spelling and syntax, inclusion of complete and correct references to bibliography and illustrations, accuracy of information as far as you know.

2. Sentence by sentence and paragraph by paragraph for clarity and succinctness. If you have to read a sentence twice in order to understand it, then it needs to be changed. You should also be alert to the possibility of libel.

3. Section by section and chapter by chapter for sense. You are looking to ensure that the author's arguments are cogent, continuing and finally conclusive, that he does not introduce a new idea or character and then abandon it or him unresolved. In other words that the book hangs together as a complete work. (Baker, 1987)

Sub-editors are the unsung heroes of the book trade. A good one can transform a mediocre manuscript into a reasonably good one but rarely gets any acknowledgement for it. The sub-editor has the difficult task of making sure that your book conforms to the publisher's 'house style' and is intelligible. On the other hand, she also has to retain the author's own style and approach to writing. Her aim is not to mechanically reduce every manuscript to a pre-determined format. If your book is well sub-edited, write and thank the sub-editor.

DEALING WITH QUERIES, THE AUTHOR'S QUESTIONNAIRE AND PROOFREADING

After the sub-editor has worked carefully through your manuscript, she will have put together a list of queries about your work. This will usually take the form of conflicting dates of references in the text and in the list at the end, unclear phraseology or (if you are lucky) queries about the accuracy of some of the statements you have made. Again, deal with these quickly but make sure that your answers are fully made and that you make it absolutely clear what you mean. Writing 'OK' next to a query is not sufficient: you must make it completely obvious what you are saying OK to.

This is the last chance you have to make modifications to your manuscript. You cannot make changes at proof stage. If you really must make changes, make them now. Don't expect the sub-editor to be pleased with you. Changes should have been made before you submitted the manuscript.

Be considerate of the sub-editor's queries. Sometimes, a point that is obvious to you is queried by the sub-editor. She is unlikely to be an expert in your particular field. If a point is not clear to the sub-editor it is unlikely to be clear to the general reader of your book. Bear in mind, though, that the sub-editor is the expert in editing. Read through any proposed changes carefully and do not dismiss them lightly. I have nearly always found that sub-editors improve on the original text. Figure 10.3 is an example of a set of sub-editor's queries and the author's response to them.

About this time, too, you will be sent an 'author's questionnaire'. This will ask you a whole range of questions about your book. You will be asked, for

Smith and Davies Ltd.

EDITORIAL QUERY SHEET

TITLE: Developing Professional Skills   Author: Edwards, J.

QUERY From sub-editor	REPLY/COMMENT from author
P24. 'Professions': should this be Professionals?	Yes.
P36. 'Lain': should this be 'Latin'?	Yes.
P67. 'of' in question: is this right? Should it be 'for'?	Yes, it should be 'for'.
P98. 'Indifference': should this be 'indifferent'?	Yes.
P125. 'can perhaps ... rather than ...: is a word missing here?	Yes, please insert 'hinder'
p240. Cooper reference: no journal title.	Journal title is Nurse Educator.
P300. Brown (1994): Initial missing.	Initial is J.
P302. Moore, Bianchi-Gray and Stevens: no initial for Stevens.	Initial is P.
P305. Yardley and Honess (1987): not in refs.	Yardley, K. and Honess, T. (eds) (1987) Self and Identity, Wiley, Chichester
P303. Smith and Cassen (1986): 1987 in refs.	1987 is correct.
P45. Saunders, not Owen in refs	Saunders is correct.
P67. Peters, 1976, 1969: 1972 in refs.	1976 is correct. Please adjust 1969 ref and remove 1972 ref.
P79. Andrews, 1958: 1957 in refs.	1957 is correct
P128. Brown, 1989: 1981 in refs	1989 is correct.
P230. Johns, 1993: a or b?	'a' is correct.
P268. Shaffer, 1978: Shafer in refs.	Shaffer is correct.
P260. Whittaker (or Whitaker over page) 1987: not in refs	Whitaker, D.S. (1987) Using Groups to Help People, Tavistock/Routledge, London.

Figure 10.3 Set of sub-editor's queries.

example, to describe the book in a sentence, a short paragraph and to list the aims of the book. Spend considerable time filling this in carefully. The information gleaned from this questionnaire helps the publisher to brief sales staff and to sell your book. It may be tedious (and, for some reason, it almost always is) but do it well. Again, do it quickly. The author's questionnaire nearly always follows the following format and it is worth considering, in advance, what your answers to some of the questions might be. The more time you investing in working through these questions, the better the publishers will be able to market your book. Don't skimp on it. The items in a typical questionnaire are these – and I have added comments on them:

1. **Title of the book**
2. **Your name, qualifications and affiliations**   Note that this will be used as text in promotional material. Decide, beforehand, whether or not you want all your qualifications next to your name or whether or not you want to be associated, directly, with your place of work. If you work in a large college, do you want to be associated, mostly, with the college, itself, or – more specifically – with the department within that college?
3. **Your nationality and date of birth**   These are required for the registration of your book's copyright.
4. **Home and work addresses and telephone numbers**   In this section, the publisher usually asks you which point of contact you would prefer. If you possibly can, quote a fax number in this section to allow the editor to get in touch with you quickly.
5. **Career and present position**   Many publishers ask for a listing of work experience in the format of a short CV. Some, too, ask you to describe yourself in a fairly short paragraph. Don't be over modest in this section. Again, the text may appear in advertising material. Obviously, though, do not make false claims about yourself.
6. **Previous publications**   List, here, any other books, journal papers or articles that you have had published.
7. **Description of the book**   Now the fun starts. In this section, you are normally asked to describe your book in about 250 words. You are required to say something about the purpose, aims, scope and general approach of the book. Again, choose your words carefully – and note the next section.
8. **Description of your book in a few sentences**   This is the condensed version and often the most difficult to write. This and the previous section are two of the most important items in the questionnaire. Take your time over them.
9. **What are the key features of your book?**   You may be having a sense of déjà vu at this point. You may feel that you have said all that you can about your book in the previous sections. Here, though, you are required to supply a 'bullet list' of the most important features that differentiate

your book from others. If there is something really new or different about your book, this is the place to say it. These points often appear on the back cover of your book as part of the blurb. Remember that readers often read the back cover when trying to decide whether or not to buy **your** book. Remember, too, next time you read the back of someone else's book, that **they** probably wrote the back cover as well as the inner contents!

10. **New edition**   If this is a second or subsequent edition of your book, you are asked, here, to identify in what ways the new edition is different.

11. **Competition**   In this section, you are asked to identify the most important – in your view – competitors in the book market. Here, you compare your book with others and make sure that the publishers know that yours is the best one on the market. The information from this section is often used by sales representatives selling your book to booksellers. Be accurate about the competition but also make sure you 'sell' your own.

12. **Superiority over other books**   This is where the publisher almost calls your bluff. You have to justify why your book is better than others. Again, you may feel that you have already done this but this is the opportunity to **really** identify the differences between your book and all the others. Do this well.

13. **Weaknesses of other texts**   The publisher allows you your own back. Identify, here, the things that make the other books in the field less saleable than yours.

14. **Readership**   In this section, you identify, as clearly as possible, the groups of people that are likely to buy your book. Before you fill this section in, read the next.

15. **Course texts**   Here, you describe what, if any, courses, your book is appropriate for. You need to be accurate here as you are asked to **name** the sorts of courses that you have in mind. Be specific. No one benefits from your writing 'all courses for health professionals' in this section. You may need to do some research to fill in this – and the previous section – properly.

16. **Countries**   If you feel that your book would sell well in other countries, this is your chance to list them. It is worth discussing, with the editor, whether or not there really is likely to be a market in other countries for your book. Do not guess at it and, again, do not use vague statements like 'all English-speaking countries'.

17. **Reviews**   In this section you list the journals in which your book might be reviewed. The publishers will use your list (and its own) to make decisions about which journals should receive a free copy of your book for review purposes. Note that this does not in any way **guarantee** that your book **will** be reviewed in those journals. Book editors of journals receive huge numbers of books and reviewers often take huge amounts of time over the writing of reviews. You will probably find that you take much

less time to review **other people's** books once you have had one of your own published. You can also list overseas journals in this section. Again, be specific and be realistic. You are unlikely to get a popular book about making friends reviewed in the *British Medical Journal* – although, you might.

18. **Professional societies** Here you list any organizations, associations, unions and so on that might help to promote your book.

19. **Conferences and exhibitions** In this section, you identify any conferences that you are likely to be presenting papers at or any exhibitions in which you may feature. Sometimes, too, you are asked to list **individuals** who might be sent a free copy of your book. Identify these people **really** carefully and don't include your mother. Well placed, free copies can help to sell your book.

20. **Any other points** In this final section, you are asked to identify any suggestions you may have for promoting your book. Once again, be realistic but do write down what you feel can be done. Unless your book is considered to be a major textbook, it is unlikely that it will be very widely advertised, on its own. It will, of course, be included in the publisher's catalogues and you may like to ask for some 'flyers' so that you can engage in a bit of self-promotion. Undue modesty rarely pays. Books have a limited bookshelf life and you may as well promote your own books as hard as you can for the life that they do have. You may not be able to send everyone you can think of a copy of your book but you could certainly send them a flyer about it. You can also include these with some of your correspondence – both home and overseas.

Finally, you will be sent two copies of the proofs when they are printed. Normally, you will receive page proofs. These are rough prints of the pages of your book and will show you what the finished product will look like. I always enjoy opening parcels of page-proofs.

If you are making an index, one of the copies of the proofs is for you to use in doing that. The other set are for proofreading.

MAKING AN INDEX

Making an index is considered, by many, to be something of an art. It probably is. The good indexer anticipates the sorts of things that people are going to look up and are restrained enough not to make the list so huge that it puts the user off. A good index can be really useful. A poor one is worse than no index at all. Two examples come to mind. First, the index that accompanies the *Writer's Handbook* is an example to anyone who plans to develop an index. On the other hand, the index to Reason and Rowan's *Human Inquiry: a sourcebook of new paradigm research* (a book that is excellent in every other respect) illustrates how not to produce an index. In that book, the word 'act' is referenced to 171 page numbers while the word 'analysis' is cited 110 times. It is fairly unlikely that many people would want to look up the word 'act' and even less likely that anyone would want to check it that number of times.

There are indexers whose full-time job it is to make indexes. There are books on the topic, there are associations of indexers and even journals on indexing. In this section, I describe how **I** make an index. I have indexed most of the books that I have written and don't claim that they are examples of the state of the art. However, the method that I describe here does work.

Bear in mind that although your word-processing program is likely to have an indexing feature, you are unlikely to be able to use it at this stage. Remember that you are working with proofs supplied by the publisher. Indexing features in word processors work to the page numbers of the files that are produced within those word processors. The page numbers in proofs will be different to those in your files. Therefore, you have little option but to make your index by hand. Here is how I do it. The method, incidentally, is based to some degree on a reading of the books about indexing and to some degree on 'making it up as I went along'. I remember that, for a long time, I could not work out **at all** how to make an index: the task seemed gargantuan and I couldn't imagine where anyone started the process. Like most things, though, indexing becomes easier (and more obvious) as you start to do it.

First, though, some preliminaries. You don't need to index every word in your book. Clearly, no one is likely to want to look up 'the' or 'that'. But nor are they likely to look up the word 'counselling' in a book about counselling. After all, the **book** is about counselling. To index every occurrence of the word 'counselling' would produce huge numbers of page entries. And this leads to the second point: limit your entries. It is rarely useful to offer more than 10 page entries for any given item and even that is probably too many. If you have 50 entries, the reader is likely to spend more time with your index than reading the book. Also, if an entry **needs** 50 page references, it is likely that the reader will **chance** upon the item in question as he looks through the book.

Next, will you cite references to **authors**? If so, will you have a separate 'author's index' and 'subject index'? The decision will depend, to a considerable degree, on the number of other writers that you refer to. If your book is full of references to other writers, then an author index may be useful. On the other hand, if you refer to only a few other writers, you could include these in a single index, along with 'subjects'.

Publishers will often indicate how long an index should be. They have to work out, when budgeting for printing, how many pages will be taken up by the index. You should note this limitation and work within it. Also, as a rule of thumb, it is a good idea to have about three index entries for every page of text. This will give you an 'average' index and, usually, a useful one.

If you decide not to make your own index, the publisher will usually arrange for this to be done for you (some publishers don't give you the option: they employ a professional straight away). If you **are** given the option to make your own index and turn it down, then you will be **charged** for the cost of a professional indexer's time. This can turn out to be expensive. While you are unlikely to be invoiced, directly, the cost will be taken off your first royalties payment. On, then, to producing the index.

Stage one

Buy yourself a couple of 'highlighter' pens of the same colour. I suggest two in case one runs out half way through your indexing. Then, sit down with the proof copy that you have set aside for indexing. Read through it very slowly and mark up each word that you want to appear in the index. This will also mean marking up 'repeats' of words. Thus, once you have decided to index the phrase 'primary care' you must then mark up every instance of it, as it appears. This sounds difficult, but as you concentrate on it, it becomes less so. You end up with a proof copy that has between three and five 'highlighter marks' on each page. Mark, also, every subheading and every chapter heading.

Stage two

Sitting at the computer keyboard, starting at page 1 of the manuscript, type in each of the highlighted words and the page number on which they appear. At this stage, don't worry about the fact that they will not be in alphabetical order. The beginning of your list is likely to look like this:

Health care professionals 2
Nursing staff 2
Doctors 2
Nursing staff 3
Measles 3
Doctors 3

Stage three

Work through the entries and work on 'alternatives'. For example, the term 'health care professionals' may also be listed as 'professionals, health care'. Make sure that you work out all the alternatives that people may look for when they are looking up a particular term. This will leave you with an extended list of words and phrases.

Stage four

Use the 'sort' feature of your word processor to put all of your entries in alphabetical order. Now you will have a completed index. Check through it, a line at a time, to make sure that everything is as it should be. Sort features in word processors sometimes do some odd things and sometimes separate numbers from words. If this happens, you may have to put your index in alphabetical order, by hand.

Stage five

Proofread your index. Check that the numbers really do match up with page numbers. Spell-check the index and then double space it. Insert page numbers at the bottom of the index pages and your index is complete. Print out three copies and send two back with the proofs of the book. Keep one copy for yourself.

This is one way of making an index. Another, more traditional way, is to use sets of (appropriately named) index cards. Here, you use a separate card for each word or phrase that you decide to use in your index. You work through the book jotting down the words and phrases on the cards and noting the page numbers as you go. You then sort the cards into alphabetical order and check each card with the proofs to check that you have identified every occurrence of the word or phrase in the proofs. Finally, you type up your index from the cards, double space the manuscript and number the pages of the index.

PROOFS

Proofs are for checking and not for changing. It cannot be stressed too strongly that you cannot make changes at this stage. If you do, you are likely to be charged for the cost of resetting the pages. Check proofs, don't change them. The publisher will send you a set of symbols to use for marking up the page proofs. Learn to use them and use them clearly. If you cannot use them, make corrections clearly both in the text itself and in the margin. Although two or three other people will also read proofs, make sure that you read them thoroughly. It does neither you nor the publishers any good if the final book is full or errors (or 'typos' as they are called). Try to read the proofs carefully but quickly. I try to return proofs the day after I receive them: if this means sitting up late, then I think it's worth it.

Finally, after another long wait and after possible consultation about the cover, you will receive a pre-publication copy of your book, followed by your free copies. This is usually the best day of all. Show it to everyone, put it on the bookshelf, take it off again and admire it and then get to work on your next proposal. Meanwhile, do what you can to encourage people to buy your book. Even better, try to get people to include it on book lists for courses. Once a book is on a book list, it usually stays there. That means that for the next two or three years, students will be buying your book. That means that you make royalties.

WAITING FOR THE REVIEWS

Once you have got over the shock of seeing your book in print, the next wait is that for reviews. Reviews usually appear between four and twelve months after publication. Sometimes, they don't appear at all. Magazines and journals receive huge numbers of books for review and cannot even print all the reviews that they get back from reviewers.

As ever, too, the silence of the publishers on matters relating to the book is deafening. In 1924, W.B. Maxwell wrote the following about that silence. He could have been writing this year.

> The silence of publishers is awful. An author, whether young or old, wants to know what happens when his new book appears, but rarely if ever does the publisher tell him. On the day of publication, not a word is said; on that day, week, that day fortnight, the same ominous silence is preserved. Another mute week passes, and the author still doesn't know if one copy or a million copies have been sold – he knows nothing until, if he is lucky, he sees an advertisement of his work saying, 'Three editions exhausted in the same number of weeks. Fourth edition binding, fifth edition printing, six edition ordered'. But even then the publisher is still silent. (Maxwell, 1924)

You hope, obviously, for a good review and they are always the best sort. Often, though, they give you a completely different insight into your own work and a well-written review can teach you something about writing. The writer Primo Levi sums up the 'different insight' position in one of his books:

> It is known that no author deeply understands what he has written and all authors have had the opportunity of being astonished by the beautiful and awful things that the critics have found in their work and that they did not know they had put there ... (Levi, 1989)

You don't usually have to scour the journals for reviews of your book (although you probably will): the publisher will probably send you a photocopy of the review after it is published. If the review is good, the publisher will also incorporate part of the review into promotional material. They may even include a short quotation from a review on the back cover of subsequent print-ings of the book. In the end, though, it is difficult to know the degree to which good or bad reviews affect the sales of non-fiction books. Fifty years ago, Clifton Fadiman, a writer and book reviewer, wrote the following and it proba-bly still applies today:

> *How influential are reviewers?* This is a hard one to answer. All the publishers' questionnaires, scientifically designed to discover just why a given book is bought, throw but a dim light on the subject, though they provide a desired quantity of statistics. Reader A buys a book because his friend B has mentioned it; that is apparently the strongest single definable

factor. But this means nothing unless you know why B happened to mention it. You ask B. B replies, let us suppose, that he himself brought, read and recommended the book as the result of reading an advertisement. Now you have to find out what in that particular advertisement caused the positive reaction to the book. Was it the publisher's statement of the book's merits? Was it a quotation from a reviewer? If the latter, B bought the book because the reviewer liked it – and therefore A indirectly did the same. The whole matter is very complex. (Fadiman, 1944)

Probably **any** review is better than no review at all – based on the old show-business saying that 'it doesn't matter what they write about you, as long as they get your name right'. The point is that a review does draw attention to your work.

If you do get bad reviews and things begin to get you down, take to heart the advice offered by the writer Doris Lessing (1984):

> it does no harm to repeat, as often as you can, 'Without me the literary agency would not exist: the publishers, the agents, the sub-agents, the sub-sub agents, the accountants, the libel lawyers, the departments of literature, the professors, the theses, the books of criticism, the reviewers, the book pages – all this vast and proliferating edifice is because of this small, patronized, put-down and underpaid person (Lessing, 1984).

Incidentally, it is almost impossible to assess, as an author (or perhaps even as a publisher) how **many** of your books will sell. Recently, one of my books on communication sold 3000 copies in a year. Another, on a similar subject, sold 7. Was one **that** much better (or worse) than the other?

SECOND EDITIONS

Make sure that you keep copies of your book manuscript on disk. If the book sells well, the publishers may ask you to write a second edition. Or you can suggest writing one. Second editions usually appear about five years after the first edition.

The writing of a second edition is often more interesting than the writing of the first. You have the chance really to get to know the book that you wrote, to correct it where necessary and to bring it up to date. The aim is not to write a completely new book. The second edition should retain the 'character' and even the layout of the first. After all, if the book is selling well, it is likely that it has become a course book in many colleges. If lecturers are using your book to augment their courses, they will want to know that a new edition is not too dissimilar to the first. It is usual to introduce about 25% new material into a second edition. It is also usual to retain the original title of the book.

Remember that if you refuse to prepare a second edition and the publishers are determined that one should be written, most book proposals contain a clause which states that, should the author refuse, the publishers may ask another author to write the second edition. If the second edition **is** written by another author and if your book has become something of a classic, your name may be retained in the title of the book. This accounts for those rather oddly titled books such as *Bacon's Textbook of Psychiatry* by Davies and Smith.

As a general rule, if you are asked to prepare a second edition, do so. Remember that you are likely to see a revival of interest in your book when the second edition comes out and that usually means an increase in sales. Sometimes, too (and for reasons that I don't understand), second editions sell better than first editions. Perhaps the phrase 'second edition', on the cover, gives the book-buying public a certain confidence that the book cannot be too bad if it has run to two editions. Also, second editions usually have new covers. If you really hated the cover of your first edition, now is the time to express an interest in the colour scheme of the new one.

Before you write the second edition, you will have to write a new proposal and show the publishers how you plan to organize the work. This proposal, like the original one, will have to be approved by a publishing committee and may be sent out for review. Do not start writing the second edition until you have a contract to do so.

If your book seems to be selling well in two editions, you may want to open a series of files on your computer into which you place new material for subsequent editions. In this way, you 'live' with your book and are constantly on the lookout for new material. Given that there is nearly always a five-year gap between editions, you are going to have plenty of time to find your new material. What is particularly useful about this 'collect as you go' approach is that it allows you to keep up to date with the **literature and research** in the field related to your book. Also, as the author of a successful book, you are likely to be invited to give talks or conference papers on the subjects in your book. Keeping up to date is therefore essential.

Note that you are unlikely to receive an advance on royalties for second and subsequent editions and all of the comments, above, apply to third, fourth and fifth editions.

EDITING BOOKS

If you are uncomfortable about writing or unable to write a whole book yourself, you may want to edit a book with contributions from other authors. This is by no means an easy option. In many ways, as we shall see, being the editor of a multi-authored work is more complicated than writing the book yourself. Sometimes, too, you end up virtually writing the whole book anyway.

There are certain advantages to an edited volume:

• the work is distributed among a number of writers;

- there is the chance to group together 'experts' in the field;
- a number of writers benefit from having their work published;
- various writers can bring variety to a book.

Be aware, though, that there are also certain disadvantages:

- those who promise chapters may pull out later on;
- contributors may change job or leave the country;
- writers may submit their chapters late;
- there may be considerable overlap in information between the chapters which will have to be edited out;
- contributions may vary, considerably, in style, quality and length;
- you may have to spend a considerable time on ensuring that the final work is consistent in style and quality.

It is sometimes tempting to draw together a group of friends or colleagues to work on an edited volume. If you do this, remember that, at a later date, you will have to read and critically comment on their work. This may or may not be a painful process. It may also be the case that certain friends and colleagues write really well and others do not. In this case, the ones who do not may wonder why you have singled them out for critical attention.

The secret to working on an edited volume, if there is one, is to **structure** the project very tightly. First, make sure that you invite only those people who you know will finish chapters and who will submit to a deadline. Second, work with all of the contributors on the book proposal. Make sure that there is as little overlap as possible and make sure that everyone knows what everyone else is writing about. Overcome any reticence you may have about asking to see potential contributors' previous work. Many people like the idea of contributing to a book but not everyone can do it. Third, prepare a set of guidelines relating to style, layout, length and so forth. Ask all contributors to stick very rigidly to these guidelines. The more structure that you can introduce at the early stages of the project, the less editing of the manuscript you are likely to have to do later on. Fourth, make sure that all contributors can send you their work on a disk and that they will be working with a word processor that is compatible with your own. You are going to have to edit the whole volume. If you cannot 'import' a particular chapter file into your word processor, you are going to have to retype it. This final point is a particularly important one. It is essential that you know, in advance, what sort of word processors your contributors are going to use. Figure 10.4 illustrates a set of notes that I and a co-editor sent to contributors to a multi-author book.

Title of the book

Authors' names (eds)

We are very pleased that you have agreed to work on this project with us and we look forward very much to your chapter.

Editorial notes

These notes have been compiled to help you write your
chapter and to help in maintaining a consistent style
in the book. We hope they will be useful. They are
only <u>guidelines</u>: don't feel too constrained by them
and do come back to us for further discussion if you
would like to modify them for your chapter.

Aim of the book

The book should be a readable and practical account
of what it is like to do counselling in various nursing settings. Your aim should be to write a fairly
personal and very practical chapter. It should not be
too academic but should be appropriately referenced
to the research and the literature. Don't feel,
though, that you must support every statement that
you make with a reference.

Market

We hope that the book will appeal to students on
Project 2000, undergraduate and counselling courses.
It should also be of value to clinical nurses, nurse
educators and managers.

References

Please use the Harvard system of referencing as in
the following example. Please make sure that all your
references are complete at the end of your manuscript.

Counselling has been widely used in intensive
care settings for helping relatives to cope with
grief (Brown 1993; Smith 1993).

Brown, N. (1993) *Counselling in Intensive Care*,
Macmillan, London.

Presentation of manuscript

We would be very pleased if you were able to submit
your manuscript to us on a 3½ disk in one of the
following formats:

● WordPerfect 5.0, 5.1 or WordPerfect for Windows;
● ASCII format. Almost all word processors can

produce ASCII files but remember that in such files all special codes (such as bold and italic) are lost.

Please do not submit on Amstrad PCW disks. If you cannot submit in one of the above formats, please send your manuscript prepared as follows:

- Double line spaced
- Printed on one side of A4 paper
- Page numbered

Don't forget to keep a copy of everything that you send to us.

Layout

Whichever of the above formats you use, please observe the following style conventions:

1. Write short sentences and short paragraphs.
2. Try to put references at the ends of sentences rather than in the middle of them.
3. Use only **one** level of subheading, in the way that we have used them in this document.
4. Paragraphing. Do not indent below a chapter heading or immediately below a subheading. Indent all subsequent paragraphs. Do not leave a further space between paragraphs. An example of a page of text, in this format, is included, below.
5. Your manuscript should be between 5000 and 6000 words in length. Please stay within these limits.

Personal details

Please include, on a separate sheet or in a separate file, the following:

- Your full name
- Your qualifications
- A one-paragraph bibliographic note that includes your present job.

Proposal

We enclose the original proposal for this book so that you can see what the other chapters will be about.

Other points

• Try to define the <u>context</u> of your chapter very early on. If you are writing, for example, about psychiatric nursing, briefly describe when and in what circumstances counselling might be used.
• You don't have to subscribe to any particular school of counselling but try to define and discuss your approach.
• If you can, offer direct, practical examples of the ideas that you are discussing.
• Do try to write the 'dialogue' section of the chapter. You can base this on your own experience or, if you have them, on taped counselling sections. Have someone else read them through to vouch for their 'realism'.
• Do try to avoid writing too much in the 'first person'. Use 'I' when you want to refer, directly, to a personal experience but avoid using it too often.

Deadline

You can either submit the final manuscript to us or you can send a draft on which we will offer comments if these are appropriate. Deadlines are as follows:

• If you are submitting a draft: 1st December 1993
• Deadline for submission of final manuscript: 1st February 1994

We plan to submit the final manuscript to (publisher) in June 1994.

We hope you will enjoy working on your chapter and we look forward to working with you on this exciting project. Do contact either or us at any time if you would like to talk through any aspect or your work.

Figure 10.4 Notes sent to contributors of a multi-author book.

The proposal for an edited volume has to be processed by the publisher in exactly the same way as a single-author book. It will be considered by a publishing committee and will be sent out for review. At this stage, of course, individual contributors' ideas may be changed by the reviewers of the proposal. At this stage, too, potential contributors may pull out of the project, having decided that the 'modified' proposal does not fall in line with their original intentions. The egos involved in multi-author books can be very fragile! If contributors do pull out of the project, it falls to you to find new ones. It is always a good idea to have a 'second team' of potential authors of chapters on whom you can call if 'first team' authors pull out.

Chapter authors of edited volumes are usually paid on a 'one-off' basis. When the book is published, each author receives a single amount in payment for his or her work. You can either negotiate this figure with the authors or stipulate what it will be. Remember that all of these one-off payments will be deducted from your royalties. You will not begin to see any royalty payments from an edited volume until all of the individual authors have been paid off.

Edited volumes usually take a long time to produce. As we have seen, individual authors can be slow to send you their manuscripts. What seemed like a good idea to them six months ago may become something of a burden as time goes by. The motivation for writing a single chapter is not usually as high as it is for writing a single-author book. It is useful to keep in touch with your authors and, if possible, to meet with them as a group about half way through the timespan allotted for the writing.

Once you have all the manuscripts in and you have converted the various word-processing formats to your own word processor, you can begin to edit. Specifically, you must edit for the following:

- overall style;
- tense and person;
- grammar and spelling;
- content;
- layout.

When the going gets tough, remember that the editor **always** has the last word. If you feel strongly that something should be changed in a particular chapter, then change it. Just as you will never be completely happy with the final product when you are working on a single-author book, so you will always find problems with contributions in a multi-author book. As I have indicated, above, you may find yourself 'rewriting' the whole of the book. If this happens, it suggests that you have not done sufficient groundwork and planning in the early stages of the project.

Once the manuscript has been sent to the publisher, it will, again, be reviewed by external reviewers. There may, again, be suggestions for change and these changes will have to be made by individual authors. Finally, proofs will have to be read. You will be asked to do an overall proof check and each author, individually, will also be asked to proofread his or her contribution. The indexing of multi-authored books is probably best left to a professional indexer. Remember: you will not 'know' the content of a multi-authored book in the way that you would a book that you wrote yourself. Personally, I would never take on the task of indexing an edited book and I have edited a few.

At the risk of sounding grim: don't take on the editing of a multi-author book lightly. Do not see it as an easy option for getting into print and don't be 'talked into it' by a group of potential authors or a publisher. Only take on such a project if you really know the field well and if you have already had some editorial experience. Each time I have taken on the editing of a multi-authored text I have sworn that it would be the last time!

WRITING REVIEWS

As you write, others will ask you to review what other people have written. There are at least four reviewing possibilities:

- book reviews;
- reviews of book proposals;
- reviews of journal papers;
- reviews of completed manuscripts.

Book reviews

Many people who work in academic departments are likely to be asked to review books for journals. If you have also published quite widely yourself, you are also likely to be asked.

The first point about book reviewing should be obvious but is not always. If you are sent a book to review, read it. It is **possible** to write a review by reading the 'blurb' on the back cover and by flicking through the chapters. This is, however, unfair to the writer, to the publisher and to the readers of the journal in which your review is to appear. The publisher and author will immediately recognize the 'blurb review'. After all, who writes the blurb? The editor or the author.

A well-crafted review is quite difficult to write. Most people can summarize the chapters and say whether or not they liked the book. The point, though, is to offer a little more than this. The reader may also **like** reading book reviews. Have a look at the Sunday papers: the large ones contain separate review supplements and they are not there simply to sell books. They are there, also, because people enjoy reading them. So your review might entertain as well as guide the potential reader.

Start, perhaps, by summarizing the book. Say in a few sentences what the book is about and whom it is aimed at. Then do a **brief** summary of the main points of the book. Close by offering an opinion on the value of the book in terms of its content, its readability and its general usefulness (or otherwise) to the potential reader.

Don't be afraid to write a 'bad' review but please remember that the author will read the review, too. As you write the review, imagine that this is **your** book. You have spent months working on it and are proud to see it in the shops.

By all means point out the bad points of the book but I see little value in really 'panning' a book. It might be better to return it to the book review editor and suggest that you don't feel that it is an appropriate book to review. This, I accept, is a contentious view. Others take the view that the reviewer should be as 'honest' as possible and as readily damn the book as to praise it. My feeling is that such an approach adds little to a book review and does not help the reader very much – accept that it might give some goulish pleasure in seeing someone else's work torn to shreds.

Work strictly to word limits when reviewing books. You may be asked to write a review of anywhere between 100 and 5000 words. Either way, it is important to keep within those limits. If you do not, the journal will either edit your review drastically or will simply not print it.

Payment for reviewing varies from nothing at all to a few pounds. No one ever made a fortune from reviewing books (unless, of course, you become a featured book reviewer in the Sunday papers). All journals that I have come across let you keep the book that you review.

Only review books that you feel capable of reviewing. Much as you may feel flattered by being asked to review a book and might like the idea of keeping this hefty textbook that lands on your desk, only do it if it falls within your own field of expertise. To do otherwise is likely to lead to an inaccurate and not very helpful review.

Not everyone, of course, thinks that book reviewing is such a great occupation. In an interview with Robert Butler, the author and humorist Stephen Fry had this to say about reviewing:

'But you wouldn't want to be the one doing it, would you?' He offers his St Peter scenario. 'Imagine getting to the gates of heaven and St Peter says 'What did you do with your life?'

'Well, I spent my life looking at things that other people did and saying "oh, I think we've seen that all before, haven't we?" And "that's not very good". And "oh dear, oh dear, oh dear".' (Butler, 1995)

Reviews of journal papers

You may be also be invited to review other people's manuscripts sent to journals. Many health care journals use a 'blind', peer review process. That is to say that the writer's name is taken off the front of the manuscript before it is sent out to two reviewers who are deemed experts in the field. The journal will usually only publish papers that are accepted by both reviewers. Note, though, that the editor always has the final say in what does and what does not get published in a journal. It is possible for two reviewers to agree that a paper is worthy of publication and for the editor to decide not to accept it. Obviously, the editor has a clearer view of what is already waiting for publication and what is in keeping with the journal's policy.

If you are sent a paper for review, you will usually be sent a form to complete that has two sections: comments to the editor and comments to the writer. You will also be asked to express a view on whether or not the editor should accept the paper for publication. In recent years, some journals have begun to send out quite detailed questionnaires to their reviewers.

As you read the paper, consider, at least, the following points:

- Is the paper similar in style to other papers published in the journal?
- Is it original and does it have 'something to say'?
- If it is a research paper, have all the stages of the research process been described properly and appropriately?
- Is the layout of the paper and the reference list appropriate and complete?
- Would you recommend publication?

Be honest and constructive in your comments to the writer. This is not a time to 'score points' or to demonstrate your own knowledge about the topic in hand. It is the chance to offer valuable feedback to another person who, like you, is struggling with the writing process. If you feel that the topic discussed in the paper is beyond your expertise, don't hesitate to send the paper back with a covering letter explaining why you feel you cannot review it.

Deal with reviews of manuscripts promptly. Editors depend on a quick turn-around of papers and writers, obviously, want to be put out of their misery as quickly as possible. Do, however, make sure that you give each manuscript enough time and read it thoroughly. If necessary, write comments directly onto the manuscript as well as on the review form. Some journals pay you for your review while others do not. Normally, the 'heavyweight' journals do not pay for reviews. Either way, you learn a great deal about writing from reading other people's work and learn a considerable amount about the right and wrong ways of preparing journal papers.

Reviews of book proposals

If you have particular expertise in a particular field, you may be asked by a publisher to review a book proposal. The publisher is likely to ring or write to you first, then send you the proposal. He or she will ask for a report that covers the following sorts of questions:

- Is there a reasonable market for a book on this topic?
- Will this sort of book have appeal in other countries? If so, which?
- Who would be the main buyers of a book like this?
- Is the author an authority in this field?
- In the case of edited books, are the contributors authorities?
- Is the contents list complete and arranged logically?
- Are there any alterations you would like to recommend?
- Which books are likely to be the main competitors with this one?

- How do you feel this book would compare with those competitors?
- Do you recommend that we should publish this book?
- Do you have any further comments?

Be fair, honest and constructive. On the one hand, the publisher will not want to publish a book that is clearly not going to sell. On the other, the potential author will appreciate constructive comments about how to improve a proposal. If you really feel that the book should not be published, outline very clearly your objections to it and the grounds for those objections. Sometimes, the publishers will send you one or more sample chapters to read and this can be a very useful indicator of the author's style. It is one thing to write a proposal and another to write the book. You are likely to receive a fee for reading and reporting on a proposal.

Reviews of completed manuscripts

If the publisher accepts yours and other reviewer's comments and offers the author a contract, the book will then be written. The publishers may then approach you again to review the whole of the manuscript. This may also happen regardless of whether or not you reviewed the original proposal.

In these cases, you need to give the manuscript a careful, line-by-line reading for style, content, consistency, readability and accuracy. The publisher is likely to ask you for a report along the following lines:

- Is there a real need for this book and what are the likely markets for it? Please indicate the level at which the book is likely to appeal and identify the likely buyers:
    in the United Kingdom;
    in the USA;
    elsewhere.
- If the book has been written for the student market, how would you anticipate its being used – as a main text, as recommended reading or as 'library only'? If you can, please list likely courses.
- What would you imagine to be a reasonable price for this book?
- What are the likely competitors for this book and how to they compare with it? What particular advantages and disadvantages has the new book?
- How quickly is it likely to become out of date?
- Is the author a recognized authority in this field?
- Is the author's coverage of the material adequate and appropriate? If not, what modifications do you feel are needed?

Read the manuscript careful and give considerable thought to your report. This is rarely the time to suggest that the manuscript needs to be rewritten from the ground up. By now, the author's proposal will have been accepted, he or she will have met with the editor and probably kept in touch with him or her throughout the writing process. The end product should be very much in line with the researched proposal. If, however, you feel that it is not, don't be afraid to say so. Again, be as constructive as possible: don't 'look' for faults but do comment on them if you find them. You will receive a fee for this work and may or may not receive a copy of the book when it is published.

You can learn a very considerable amount from reading other people's proposals and manuscripts. They can teach you about other people's perceptions of the field and about how other people construct books. What you clearly cannot do, however, is to 'borrow' ideas from them. Remember that whatever another person writes, it is copyright from the moment it is written. It does not have to be formally 'published' to make it copyright.

CONCLUSION

This chapter has identified the bones of book and review writing. I hope that it has demonstrated that writing a book is possible if you structure the process. I think it is one of the more enjoyable activities in life: I hope you will too.

Finally, a plea for sanity. The most important issue in non-fiction writing is the **content**. Many people find that they are so worried about **style** that they do not get as far as addressing the content. Sometimes, the style gets in the way and makes unclear what the content is. Start, then, with your content. Work out what it is you want to say and then write it down. I have used this method a lot with students who are worried about how to write a particular passage. I ask them to **tell** me what they want to write. When they have spoken, I suggest that they write down what they have said. This is nearly always the best way to write. If you can say it, you can write it.

Your aim is not to be the Joseph Conrad of essay, book and project writing. It is to convey your ideas to other people. If you stick to the basic rules of writing suggested in this book and keep your sentences and paragraphs short, you will already be some way towards effective writing.

Perhaps it is true that self-delusion most often takes the form of a belief that one can write; as to that I cannot say. My own experience has been that there is no field where one who is in earnest about learning to do good work can make such enormous strides in so short a time.

Dorothea Brande

So much for the theory. How does it all work in practice? In this chapter, I offer an illustration of the way that I write. Some books start with an introduction to the author. This one ends with one. I hope that the chapter helps to consolidate some of the issues that I have discussed in the text and also show how, in the end, there are no, immutable, rules of writing. In the end, you have to find your own way. The rules, though, can help early on in structuring and making it possible to get decent marks in assignments, get articles and books published and hand in reasonable theses and research reports. Many people don't write at all because they don't know where to start.

I have been writing for publication for ten years. During that time I have written various books – some of which have been translated into various languages – over 200 articles and papers for journals and various research reports, educational documents and many book and software reviews.

My first book was written longhand on a series of A4 pads and I found myself absorbed in the task. It took about 6 months to complete and then the handwritten manuscript was typed out by someone else. Ever since then, I have always written books on a computer and would not recommend to anyone writing a book in longhand – unless you have plenty of time and plenty of money for the typing up.

Writing the first book made the process of writing articles and papers seem easier and I went on to write more. I have also been fortunate in being asked to review other people's book proposals and their completed manuscripts. This is to be recommended. Seeing how other people work gives you lots of ideas about your own style.

EQUIPMENT AND ENVIRONMENT

I'm not fussy where I write. I have never found the need to be cloistered and to shut myself away to work. Much of my writing is done in the sitting room or dining room of our house. Other work I do on the move, while travelling. Computing seems, to me, to have made a difference to all this. Their portability and the fact that you can quickly switch them on and off means that you don't, necessarily, have to set aside a 'writing area'. Besides, we don't have the room. I have written over a period that exactly matches the growing up of my two children and I have got used to them – and various pets – being around while I work. An important point is that they can also draw you **away** from work. As far as computing is concerned, this is a good thing. It is far too easy to sit in front of a screen for far too long. Having said that, I find I write best at night and often sit up very late to finish particular projects.

At the time of writing, I have four computers. Two are both 486s with 8 mb of RAM and large hard disks. One is a desktop model and the other is a notebook. The third computer is a palmtop and the fourth is an Amstrad Notepad. The last is something of a hybrid. It is about the size of an A4 notebook, weighs only a few pounds and runs on batteries for about 40 hours. It has no hard disk or even floppy drive. Everything is stored in memory and it can only store about 12 pages of text. It is possible, though, to buy plug-in memory cards that will store considerably more. It has a full-size keyboard and is ideal for working on while travelling. After use, all work is transferred to an IBM compatible machine for further editing.

I also have a laser printer that I use to print out the final manuscript. Nothing gets onto paper before the final manuscript is finished. I don't find it useful to make lots of 'hard' (or paper) copies of things I have written and I don't keep hard copies of articles that I have sent off for publication. I do, however, keep a hard copy of book manuscripts. This is so that any editors' queries can be dealt with promptly and direct from the page. The editor, for example, sends a list of queries and all of them relate to particular pages of a manuscript. Checking these against a 'computer copy' can be difficult as page numbers sometimes get changed in the process. Working with a hard copy makes the work easier.

I find myself using the desktop computer less and less (and did not use it at all for this edition of this book). The notebook computer, although it has an inferior screen, has all the advantages of such machines. It is light and portable, can be used while sitting half-watching television and generally keeps me in the middle of things in terms of family life. The palmtop computer is ideal for working when travelling – particularly on planes and trains. While it is possible to use a notebook computer in these conditions, you have to be pretty extrovert to do so. The palmtop – a Psion series 3a – is tiny but has a usable keyboard and the files produced with it can be transferred to the notebook or desktop computer. It has the added advantage of running for up to 80 hours on a set of AA batteries and this means it can be used throughout a long-haul flight as well as on longer train journeys without the certain knowledge that the batteries will go flat. At the moment, my notebook computer will only run for about 3 hours before the battery runs out.

I use a very limited number of programs – having tried out and reviewed a great number. My word processor is Word for Windows and I also use the freeform database program Idealist for storing bibliographical references. I find the combination of the two particularly useful. When I am working on an article or a book, I have both of them running under Windows. Then, when I need a reference, I can switch from Word for Windows, into Idealist, look up the reference and then use 'copy and paste' features to transfer the reference from the database to the word processor. Over the years I have used various methods of storing bibliographical references but have found this to be the easiest and most accessible. Oddly enough, some of the most awkward programs to use are the **dedicated** referencing programs. I've never found them to have the flexibility of Idealist.

Idealist is also the program I use for collecting material for books. Its 'freeform' nature means that I can store quotations, ideas, passages of text and so on, all together in the same database. Later, I can pull out the various entries that I want as I work on the book. If I know that I will be doing a second or subsequent edition of a book, I start collecting material in this way when preliminary discussions have taken place with the publishers. If nothing comes of the idea for a new edition, I can always use the material in other ways.

The other programs that I use are PC Tools and PowerPoint. PC Tools is a set of applications that can get you out of various fixes. The program can defragment your hard disk, check for viruses, manage your files and so one. Most importantly, though, it can rescue your work when something dreadful happens. Recently, I had a hard disk 'crash' on my computer at work and found, to my considerable discomfort, that I did not have an up-to-date backup of all of the work on it. (Since then, everything – everything – gets backed up to a tape streamer on all machines.) When the crash occurred, PC Tools was the program that got me out of a fix. First, I used an 'Emergency Disk' that PC Tools makes for you for use on such occasions. This got the computer started. Next, the programs on the emergency disk went to work in various ways. One program rewrote the BIOS of the computer so that the hard disk could be recognized, another ran a 'disk-fix' routine that allowed me to get most of my files back.

The process took a long time and I wouldn't wish the event on anyone but I have subsequently met lots of people to whom this has happened and, as all the computer books say, it is not a question of **if** your hard disk crashes but **when**. Backups, although tedious, have since become a regular feature of the way I work. I have always kept two copies of every book manuscript I have written on two separate disks. The thought of losing a whole manuscript is too much to think about.

PowerPoint allows me to make various visual aids and graphical items. I use it for preparing Overhead Projection Acetates, for lecturing. I also use it for preparing graphs and other charts for research reports. Such charts can be readily copied into Word for Windows – although the word processor also has its own, excellent, charting facility and sometimes I use that.

I have customized Word for Windows considerably. First, I have got rid of a lot of the buttons at the top of the screen that I don't use and replaced them with buttons that I can. I have a button for counting words, another for double spacing manuscripts, others that bring up standard templates and so on. All of these things can be done from menus but I find the buttons easier to use. Also, making buttons is something that can be done during periods of lack of inspiration, while writing. It's not difficult to convince yourself that you are doing something useful when fiddling with the features of a program.

As I write, I count words. This serves two functions. First, it convinces me that I really am making progress. I used to keep a running tally of the words I had written on given days and in this way formed a view of how well (or otherwise) I was doing. Laterally, though, I find I am better at judging how much or how little I have written and better at pacing myself. I used to be a person who had to get things done as quickly as possible – a 'type A' personality, if you like. Illness and a tendency to burnout have meant that I have slowed down and learned to be a bit more moderate in my writing habits. The second reason for counting words is to make sure that I am within the word allocation afforded by publishers or journal editors. It's no use sending in a journal paper of 6000 words when the limit is 2500.

One of the real high spots in writing is edging up towards the final word limit of a book manuscript. Sometimes, however, the anticipation of it causes a sudden drop off of inspiration. It's a bit like being an athlete and seeing the tape in front of you and suddenly feeling your legs buckling. If I sense this happening, I use rather elaborate ploys to pretend that I am not 'really' nearing the target. I stop counting words or I treat the final section as though it were an essay on its own. Or I practise 'thought blocking' if I find myself thinking about the last few thousand words. Generally the first and last two thousand words of any book are the most difficult ones to write.

THE WRITING ROUTINE

First, it **is** a routine. I try to write something every day and aim at finishing something for publication at least every month. In between times, there are various other writing projects, some work-related and others to do with reviews of books and manuscripts. I am quite sure that I would not want to be a full-time writer. It is the 'other' work that I do that feeds the writing and I can't imagine what it must be like to get up and come downstairs to a cold computer every morning. Teaching and travelling I find particularly rewarding in relation to writing. Both spark off new ideas and encourage the seeing of things from different perspectives.

When writing articles, I usually write the whole thing in my head, before sitting down at the keyboard. I rarely write 'commissioned' pieces and find these difficult. Instead, most of the articles that I write stem from ideas that I have thought about while working. Very often, the 'whole' of the plan for an article – and sometimes for a book – arrives in one 'lump'. Then, it is a question of teasing out the various points, working out headings and subheadings and deciding on whom the piece should be aimed at. I have found it useful to learn about the various house styles of different publications and then work on an article with that publication in mind. I also try to imagine the readership of a given piece although this is such an abstract idea that I am not sure that it really works.

Once I have the piece written in my head, I transfer it to the computer. I write quickly, at first, and don't stop to correct mistakes. The first draft is always a sort of 'stream of consciousness' piece, although as time has gone on, I have found it easier to structure the writing as it goes into the computer. Sometimes, I write down a series of headings before I start but, more often, I return to put the headings in later. Even in the first draft I make sure that there are lots of paragraphs breaks and use the layout of the notebook computer to help in this respect. If I have been writing for some time and cannot see any paragraph breaks on the part of the screen that is visible, I go back and insert some. It seems to me that short sentences and short paragraphs really are the basis of effective writing.

Once I have written the first draft of an article, I spell-check it. I never used to be any good at spelling but, ironically, the spell-checker has made me a better one. By being presented, on a regularly basis, with the same old errors of spelling, I have begun to absorb the correct spellings. Now, I try to beat the spell-checker.

The spell-checker takes care of some of the grosser problems with the original draft. Next, I work through the paper, a paragraph at a time, and rework each one. This is the stage, too, in which I put in references. During the writing of the first draft, I merely leave two open brackets ( ), to indicate where references should go. I always try to make sure that references go at the ends of sentences so that the reader is not distracted by a sudden outpouring of odd names and dates. The insertion of references often leads to new ideas for certain paragraphs or sections. Recalling what other writers or researchers have said leads, often, to further debate about particular issues.

I try to make the second draft the final one. The idea that your work necessarily improves the more you work on it doesn't seem to match my experience. I have found it possible to 'polish to death' a piece of writing and thus remove any sort of spontaneity or life from it. After all, the process is not a scientific one and I don't believe that you can continue to hone down a piece of writing until it approaches the ideal. All writing is something of a compromise and, looking back, I realize that some pieces I have written have been more of a compromise than others. In the end, though, it doesn't pay to be too hard on yourself. Most of us are not in the business of producing works of art. The main thing, presumably, is to communicate ideas to others in as clear a way as possible. To this end, and in the second draft, I further check sentence and paragraph length and insert headings if they are not already there. I also try to take out big words and lighten the more leaden passages. I also trim out as many of the 'howevers' and 'there is a sense in whiches' as I can find. Most writing benefits from trimming in this way.

Sometimes, I run the grammar-checking feature of the word processor. This checks for, at least, the following: spelling, tense, overly-long sentences, basic errors of grammar. It also offers a summary of the 'readability' of the text. I don't use this as a matter of course but when I am working on something very different or new or when I am writing for a particular journal that requires a particular style. Sometimes, too, the thesaurus feature of the word processor can be useful in finding alternative words.

The last thing I do with articles is to make sure that they are double-line spaced (although I work in single-line spacing 'on the screen'), page numbered and have a title page. I also pay a lot of attention to the general layout of the words on the page. I never use 'justified right' margins but leave them 'ragged' as this makes manuscripts easier to read. I also make sure that the spacing between headings and text is uniform and check, again, for typos. Obviously, spell-checkers can miss some less obvious errors such as the inappropriate uses of 'two', 'to' and 'too'.

I used to ask my wife to read articles before I sent them off but do not do so now. About five years ago she got fed up with reading them. Instead, I sometimes ask work colleagues to read them through and then make some changes. If I do this, I make them copies and ask them to write their comments directly onto the appropriate pages. This makes it easier to sit at the computer keyboard and make changes directly to the text.

Like everyone else, the articles that I send off are either accepted, rejected out of hand or sent back for modification. I try to deal with the last as soon as possible and always send a covering letter enumerating the changes that have been made. This is done in the probably erroneous belief that the editor will be pleased that I have made exactly the changes that were asked for. My experience with editors is that it mostly pays to do what you are told. Either that, or the editor can reject your work. In arguing, you may have scored on some sort of point of principle but you don't get to see your paper in print.

WRITING BOOKS

Books take much more structuring than do articles. You can't just sit down at a blank screen and start typing page one – at least, not a non-fiction book. When planning a book, again, I usually find that the idea for the book 'arrives' as a whole. Then, in my head, I separate out the various chapters. For a book of about 50 000 words, I usually aim at ten chapters and this becomes 12 or 14 for a book of up to 100 000 words. I work out a fairly detailed book proposal, including a rationale for the book, a review of some competing books, details of the various chapters and information about when the manuscript will be delivered and how long it will be. I then send it to an editor at a publisher and often I will have discussed it with that editor before I send it off. As is the case with articles, the response is the same: outright rejection, outright acceptance or acceptance subject to major or minor changes. This time, though, there are a couple of stings in the tail.

First, the proposal is sent out, by the editor, to various reviewers and this process can take a long time. By the time the reviews come in, it is sometimes possible to have rethought your position about a particular book that you have planned. Fortunately, new ideas can usually be incorporated into the manuscript.

Second, the reviewers review anonymously. That gives some reviewers licence to say exactly what they think about a proposal and some don't mince words at all. You can usually tell, from the editor's covering letter that comes to you with the reviewer's comments, that there are some 'bad' ones. In these cases, the editor will often write something like 'Don't be too put off by some of the comments: I feel that they are meant constructively.' I always am put off by them, though. It has taught me, if nothing else, to be careful what I write when reviewing other people's proposals.

Either way, if there are lots of negative responses to a proposal, the editor will, rightly, have to decide whether or not to accept a proposal or to ask for very radical changes. It isn't an exact science, though. I had one proposal turned down outright by one publisher. I then sent a very slightly modified version of it to another publisher, a year later. The second publisher offered me a contract and the book went on to sell more than any of my other books.

Early on, it was common to be invited out to lunch by the editor who would talk about your proposal and generally say pleasant things to you. This has changed in recent years although editors continue to be an approachable lot. Sometimes, if you threaten to come to London to visit them, they, in return, threaten to take you out to lunch.

Once a proposal has been accepted, a contract follows. Despite all the books saying that you should work very carefully through every clause, I rarely do this. That is not to say that I don't **read** the contract but I certainly don't send it to 'readers' for a thorough vetting. I have yet to be offered a dubious contract although I have met people who have signed contracts for very small royalty percentages. I have found the average to be 10% of the cover price. Advances are quite another thing and I have never really puzzled out the formula that is used to calculate them. When I have been with an editor who assesses the advance, they invariably do all sorts of quick calculations on the back of an envelope, narrow their eyes and then quote a figure. I am never sure that the figure they quote relates, directly, to the back-of-the-envelope work. But it may do. It is important, of course, not to be too greedy. You don't get **given** an advance: you have to earn it back in sales after the book has been published. I always forget this and I am always disappointed by the first royalty check for a new book.

Incidentally, writing non-fiction books of the sort that I write does not generate a huge, second income. I believe that the only writers who really make money out of books are the 'big names' who write potboilers. Some of the books that I have written – as research monographs – earn no royalties at all, but this is the nature of the contract with that particular publisher. One thing is essential: that all royalty statements and payment advice slips from publishers are kept for tax purposes. A good year, in royalties terms, means a bad year, the following year when the tax has to be paid. Tax returns are prepared every April and the tax bill is paid in the January and July of the following year.

Some manuscripts have to be submitted as 'camera-ready copy': what you see on the page is what I have typed on my computer. This process is painfully intense but gets easier the more you do it. The publishers that ask for copy to be prepared in this way lay down very particular standards for margin settings, page numbering, indexing and so on.

WRITING THE BOOK

Once a contract has been received and signed, I prepare the complete outline of the book in the following way. The process has become something of a ritual. First, I open up a new directory on a computer. The directory, for this book, is called 'write'. Then, I open up a series of new files, within that directory, to correspond to each of the chapters and sections of the book. Thus, apart from files for the chapters, there will be files for references, a bibliography and any appendices that are planned. In each of these files, I prepare the chapter heading and – as far as possible – all the main subheadings. I also set up any 'macros' or computerized short-cuts that will be useful during the writing of the book. Macros can be a useful way of making sure that all parts of the book are uniform. With this book, for example, I set up a macro (attached to a 'button' at the top of the screen) which prints a box on the screen for the quotations that appear throughout the book.

The structuring of an outline in this way and the preparation of the computer is an important part of the writing process. It gives me confidence that I really can finish the book and it gives me an idea of where everything is to go and what sections need further research.

At this time, I also prepare a series of envelope files to correspond to each of the proposed chapters. I use these to file away odd notes, photocopies of articles and anything else that will be useful. I mark these up with a thick marker pen to indicate the chapter number and the title of the chapter. In this way, I can quickly pull out the appropriate file. I would like to be able to say that these are then neatly filed away but they are not. They sit on the printer or – more usually – on the floor, until the book is finished. Obviously, not everything gets used but it becomes tempting to adopt a squirrel approach during the writing of a book. The other pile that tends to develop is a pile of books that becomes bigger as the book progresses. Towards the end of a book, I tend to find that I have received more than my fair share of 'overdue books' notices from various libraries. These three sources of information: the envelope files containing papers, the Idealist database containing notes and the pile of books tend to be the most frequently referred to sources during writing.

The computer files can be brought together, at any time, in Word for Windows, using the feature **masterfile**. This is a file that can automatically draw together all the other files so that it is possible to see what the whole book will look like. It is also useful, of course, when printing out the final manuscript. Incidentally, WordPerfect for Windows has a similar but much better masterfile feature.

Over the next few months, the book gets written. I work on it most days and 'live' with it all the time. I am reminded of a friend who was having psychoanalysis and who found himself dealing with the topic of 'anxiety' during one period of his analysis. During that period, he talked of nothing else. Similarly, when I am working on a book on a particular topic, I find myself caught up in noticing anything to do with that topic that appears in the press or on television. Fortunately, I have not yet got to the stage when it also becomes the only topic of conversation.

I tend to work for long periods once I get going. If I hit a real purple patch I can find myself sitting at the computer for four or five hours at the weekends. This is not to be recommended and I am working on cutting this down. Not only can it lead to problems with wrist joints but it's not particularly good for the circulation, either. It is particularly bad for family life.

I spell-check at the end of every session and word count. I also make double backups of everything. First, I back up any new work to the tape streamer. Second, I back up the chapters to a single floppy disk. Since the major hard disk crash, this is something I never skimp on. Most people have heard of horror stories in which people lost the whole of a PhD thesis from a computer and I have no particular desire to join their ranks with a book manuscript though I have lost whole chapters early in my computer career.

I don't necessarily write the chapters in the order in which they appear in the book. I tend to start with an 'easy' chapter in order to get started. Then I try to get the difficult ones written while I am still reasonably fresh. I like to finish on an easy one although the last things written are usually the conclusion and the introduction. The main difficulty is always retaining a consistency in writing style and trying not to repeat yourself. It is also important that chapters are roughly the same length and have roughly the same number of sub-sections. I also think that it is helpful to have about the same number of references at the end of each chapter.

Once the whole, draft manuscript is completed, in chapter form, I bring all the chapters together in one big file. From then on, I work with the whole manuscript. This is not as difficult as it sounds as I make a lot of use of the 'bookmark' feature of Word for Windows. The program allows you to insert labelled bookmarks at any point in the manuscript. These bookmarks can then be accessed, instantly, from a menu that can be pulled up on the screen. I make a bookmark for each of the chapter headings and then add others as the need arises. Working with the whole manuscript seems to increase the likelihood of consistency in style and layout.

There comes a point when you have to stop. The tendency is to want to keep working on a manuscript, feeling that there must be numerous ways in which it could be improved. There **are**, of course, but just sitting looking at the thing for months on end and tinkering with it are not going to guarantee quality. At some point, you decide the book is finished. Then, there are numerous checks.

The first check is for layout. Here, all the chapter headings and subheadings are checked for font size, emphasis and spacing. This may be overkill but I am a bit obsessive about such things. The second check is for the references. I run a 'search' command on an open bracket [( ] and this takes me to each reference in turn. Using the 'split' feature of Word for Windows, in which two parts of the same document can appear on the screen at the same time, I check each reference against the reference list at the end of each chapter or at the end of the book. The third check is the reference list, itself. I make sure that all the references are in the correct format and that book titles and journal titles are italicized. I also check that publishers and place of publication are complete.

Finally, the whole manuscript gets a final, on screen read through and edit and then gets printed out. I print three copies: two for the publisher and one for keeping for checking the editors 'queries'. Then, the two copies go off to the publisher in a large padded bag.

There is a sense of let down on completion of the manuscript. Having lived with it for a number of weeks or months, there is a bit of a gap and a long wait. The publisher, during this time, has sent the manuscript out to a referee to read and comment on it. It is unusual to be asked to do major surgery on the manuscript after this reading but it can happen. Once the referee has commented, the book goes to a sub-editor who checks the whole manuscript for style, consistency, spelling, grammar and so on. All of these stages are described in previous chapters of the present book. Out of all this comes the list of 'editor's queries'. These are a list of questions that relate to problems or omissions that have been highlighted during the sub-editing of the manuscript. Reading through this query list is always dispiriting: you tend to hope that you have covered most of them during your own checking of the manuscript. The truth, usually, however, is that a good sub-editor will throw up four, five or even more pages of queries. The worst are questions about missing or mixed-up dates of references. It is not uncommon to find that you have put one date in the body of the text and another in the reference list. The task, then, is to find out which is the correct one. This can mean further trips to the library as, at this point, you always doubt your memory and your ability to store references correctly in the database.

Answers to editors' queries can sometimes throw up a second list of queries. Once the sub-editor has seen your answers, he or she sometimes (and appropriately) asks 'if you have said **this** on page 34, can you say **that** on page 89? Please clarify.' Sub-editors' queries are always terse and always remind me of teacher's notes on the bottom of school essays. One day, a sub editor is going to write 'see me' at the bottom of a list of queries. For all that, a lot can be learned from responding to these queries and a lot more from seeing the sub-editor's final marking-up of the manuscript. Much of what was originally written has been crossed out, changed or rewritten in some way and nearly always (in my experience) for the better.

The relationship between a sub-editor and a writer is a strange one. While I have received letters from them, lists of queries and phone calls, I have yet to **meet** one. It is like having a slightly detached pen friend: the relationship, though, is short and sometimes intense.

Another long wait and then the proofs come for correction. I try to deal with these by return although, also due at this time, is the index. I have explained in the text how an index is prepared and it is a process that I quite enjoy. I don't enjoy proofreading, though, and I suspect that I am not very good at it. On the other hand, it is not a job to be skimped. Nor is it a task that anyone else is likely to take on for you: for love or money.

Finally, the book comes out. Sometimes, I will have had a glimpse of this before it happens. Some publishers negotiate on issues of cover colour and design. Others don't. Then, the first you know of what a book will look like is when you open the copy that is sent to you. On rare occasions, the book gets into the shops before you are sent a copy and then you have to have a good look at it there.

Then, the longest wait of all: waiting for reviews. Sometimes, of course, there aren't any. At least that saves you from the bad ones. For some reason or other, I always seem to find reviews in journals on the shelves of W. H. Smith's. If the reviews are less than glowing, I'm depressed for the rest of the day. How actors go back on stage after a night of bad notices, I don't know. On the other hand, a good review can leave you manic for a week. The worst, possibly, are the ones that are simply a summary of the blurb on the back cover. If you write reviews, please remember that the **author** also reads them. I know, traditionally, that everyone is supposed to be very adult and objective about this and no one wants a bad book to get a good review, but – please – just chose your words carefully. You're treading on someone's keyboard, as it were.

This, then, is how I write. It may not suit you. It doesn't always suit me. Nor does it do to **stick** to a routine. Every so often it is important to experiment a little and to do things differently. My aim is to write a novel. A colleague once remarked that my books already contain enough fiction. Good luck with your own writing.

Conclusion

12

It is a commonplace that every writer must turn to himself to find most of his material.

Dorothea Brande

This book has been about all aspects of the writing process. In this last chapter, I have attempted to summarize the important points about any sort of writing.

- **Use structure** Structure the way in which your work is written (by using headings and subheadings). Also structure the way you work. Break down larger projects into sections, use time in an organized way and limit the amount of time you sit and write. Don't attempt to write large projects at one sitting.
- **Remain simple in your writing** This has been a theme all the way through this book and it remains as a closing one. It is far better to keep your writing simple – whatever the project. Simple writing is better in both academic work and in the process of writing novels. Use short sentences and paragraphs, do not use complicated punctuation, avoid Latin and other 'foreign' words where possible and make sure that any reader will **understand** what you have written.
- **Keep a reference system** You must have a database that contains references to other authors' work. This can be a card file or a computerized system. Whatever system you use, keep it up to date. Do not rely on your memory, alone. Make backups of your reference files if you use a computerized system.
- **Use a computer with which to write** Once you have learned to use a word-processing package, write directly to the computer. Do not write your work out longhand and then transfer it to the computer. Instead, write quickly to the computer and edit slowly once you have written the bulk of your project.
- **Use the spell-checker** and, if in doubt, the grammar checker in your word-processing package. Both, ironically, will help to improve your spelling and grammar.

- **Count words** Whatever the project, make sure that you know how many words you have written. Checking them as you write will act as a reinforcer: every time you write a bit more, you will be nearer your target. Most writing projects involve writing to a certain limit. If you are writing for publication or a dissertation or thesis, it is **vital** that you do not exceed these limits.
- **Make sure that you read** As was noted at the beginning of this book, other people's words are the fuel for your own. Read widely, read novels and do not simply stick to the work that has been published in your own discipline. If you are a nurse, read medical journals. If you are an occupational therapist, read nursing journals and so on. Read posters, packets and newspapers. Read for style as well as for content. In particular, get to know about various journals' and publishing companies' **house styles**.
- **Pay attention to layout** A well-laid-out essay, manuscript or thesis can make a considerable 'psychological' difference to the reader. This is not to say that good layout can cover up bad work but to note that a well-produced piece of work is generally easier and more pleasurable to read. Keep the layout simple and structured and use one (or at the most, two) types of font or typeface. If you are preparing essays, manuscripts, dissertations or thesis, make sure that you double-line space your work.
- **Use diagrams and figures sparingly** Make each one earn its keep. In particular, do not be tempted to present the findings of quantitative research as a series of tables, unlinked by prose. Most people get 'number blind' very quickly. Choose the right sort of diagram or figure to represent what it is you are trying to convey. Remember, too, that diagrams and figures should be used **in place** of prose: they should, as far as possible 'speak for themselves'.
- **Practise writing** If you can, write every day. If not, write regularly and notice the development of your own style. Ask other people for feedback on your work. If you write for publication you will get this anyway. Be prepared to feel quite sensitive about reading other people's comments about your work but note what they have to say and then get back to writing.

Appendix A:
Clichés

Here is a list of clichés: health-related and otherwise. Whatever you do, lean over backwards to avoid them, like the veritable plague. Then re-read this book and see how many you can find.

A different ball game
Actual (as in 'That was an actual example of ...'
Actually
Amazing
At the end of the day
At this moment in time
Awareness
Basically
Caring for the carers
Celebration
Client-centred
Conspicuous by its absence
Downsizing
Facilitate
Gutted (as in 'He was absolutely gutted when he heard the news ...')
Had a good night (in relation to a patient or client)
Had a good day (in relation to a patient or client)
Hopefully (as in 'Hopefully, we will all be able to go home, then ...')
However
In this day and age
In the event of
In a manner of speaking
Lean over backwards
Lifestyle
Like the plague
Loved ones

May I share something with you?
Massive (as in 'he had a massive coronary')
Meaningful
Name of the game
No way (as in 'There was no way that I was going to do that ...')
Notion
On a level playing field
Open up a dialogue
Oriented
Overkill
Patient-centred
Proliferation
Quantum leap
Related (as in 'It was mostly a hospital-related service ...')
Scenario
Sick as a parrot
Simplistic
Student-centred
Superb
Target (as in 'It is terribly important that we really target all the students')
Tender loving care
The bottom line
The way forward
There is a sense in which
Throwing the baby out with the bath water
Total quality management
Track record
Very real
Viability
With all due respect

Now, add your own clichés to this list and notice how often you and other people use them – both in speech and in writing.

Appendix B: Proofreading marks

When marking proofs, all marks are best made in ink, using the following colour scheme:

Red
Errors introduced by the typesetter and to be corrected at his expense.

Blue
Author's alterations (AA) required, which may be charged extra.

Green
Comments, corrections noted by the typesetter's reader, and marked on the proofs before they are sent out.

Note that corrections to photoset matter are normally carried out in one of two ways:

a: The operator sets line or patch corrections, which are then pasted or stripped in by hand on the CRC/film by a make-up artist.

b: The operator recalls the text from file on a visual display unit, makes the correction required on the screen, and regenerates a new page/part of a page.

Each of these routes requires a completely different production process. The second is increasingly used.

The proofreading marks on the following pages are extracts from BS 5261 : Part 2 : 1976. They are reproduced with permission from BSI. Complete copies can be obtained by post from BSI Customer Services, 389 Chiswick High Rd, London W4 4AL. The marks alone are also available on a fold-out card: BS 5261 C.

INSTRUCTION	TEXTUAL MARK	MARGINAL MARK
Correction is concluded	None	/
Leave unchanged	- - - - - - - under characters to remain	✓ (circled)
Remove extraneous marks	Encircle marks to be removed	✕
Push down risen spacing material	Encircle blemish	⊥
Refer to appropriate authority anything of doubtful accuracy	Encircle words affected	(?)
Insert in text the matter indicated in the margin	⋏	New matter followed by: ⋏
Insert additional matter identified by a letter in a diamond	⋏	Followed by, for example: ⟨A⟩
Delete	/ through character(s) or ⊢——————⊣ though words to be deleted	♂
Delete and close up	through character or through characters eg chara‌cter chara‌cter	(close up ear mark)
Substitute character or substitute part of one or more word(s)	/ through character or ⊢——————⊣ through word(s)	New character or new word(s)

INSTRUCTION	TEXTUAL MARK	MARGINAL MARK
Wrong fount. Replace by character(s) or correct fount	Encircle characters to be changed	
Change damaged characters	Encircle character(s) to be changed	
Set in or change to italic	―――― under character(s) to be set or changed	
Set in or change to capital letters	≡≡≡≡ under character(s) to be set or changed	
Set in or change to small capital letters	══ under characters to be set or changed	
Set in or change to capital letters for initial letters and small capital letters for the rest of the words	≡ under initial letters and ══ under the rest of the word(s)	
Set in or change to bold type	～～～ under character(s) to be set or changed	
Set in or change to bold italic type	～～～ under character(s) to be set or changed	
Change capital letters to lower case letters	Encircle character(s) to be changed	
Change small capital letters to lower case letters	Encircle character(s) to be changed	
Change italic to upright type	Encircle character(s) to be changed	

INSTRUCTION	TEXTUAL MARK	MARGINAL MARK
Invert type	Encircle character to be inverted	
Substitute or insert character in 'superior' position	/ through character or ⟨ where required	 under character eg ^{2}
Substitute or insert character in 'inferior' position	/ through character or ⟨ where required	 over character eg $_{2}$
Substitute ligature eg fl for separate letters	through characters affected	 eg f̂l̂
Substitute separate letters for ligature		Write out separate letters
Substitute or insert full stop or decimal point	/ through character or ⟨ where required	
Substitute or insert colon	/ through character or ⟨ where required	
Substitute or insert semi-colon	/ through character or ⟨ where required	;
Substitute or insert comma	/ through character or ⟨ where required	,

INSTRUCTION	TEXTUAL MARK		MARGINAL MARK
Substitute or insert apostrophe	/ or ⋏	through character / where required	⌐
Substitute or insert single quotation marks	/ or ⋏	through character / where required	⌐ and/or ⌐
Substitute or insert double quotation marks	/ or ⋏	through character / where required	⌐ and/or ⌐
Substitute or insert ellipsis	/ or ⋏	through character / where required	. . .
Substitute or insert leader dots	/ or ⋏	through character / where required	(⋯)
Substitute or insert hyphen	/ or ⋏	through character / where required	⊢⊣
Substitute or insert rule	/ or ⋏	through character / where required	⊢
Substitute or insert oblique	/ or ⋏	through character / where required	(/)
Start new paragraph	⌐		⌐
Run on (no new paragraph)	⌒		⌒

INSTRUCTION	TEXTUAL MARK	MARGINAL MARK
Transpose characters or words	between characters or words, numbered where necessary	
Transpose a number of characters or words	3 2 1	123
Transpose lines		
Transpose a number of lines		3 2 1
Centre	Enclosing matter to be centred	[ ]
Indent		
Cancel indent		
Set line justified to specified measure	and/or	
Set column justified to specified measure		
Move matter specified distance to the right	enclosing matter to be moved to the right	
Move matter specified distance to the left	enclosing matter to be moved to the left	

INSTRUCTION	TEXTUAL MARK	MARGINAL MARK
Take over character(s), word(s) or line to next line, column or page		
Take back character(s), word(s) or line to previous line, column or page		
Raise matter	over matter to be raised under matter to be raised	
Lower matter	over matter to be lowered under matter to be lowered	
Move matter to position indicated	Enclose matter to be moved and indicate new position	
Correct vertical alignment		
Correct horizontal alignment	Single line above and below misaligned matter eg misaligned	
Close up. Delete space between characters or words	Delete space	
Insert space between characters	between characters affected	
Insert space between words	between words affected	

INSTRUCTION	TEXTUAL MARK	MARGINAL MARK
Make space appear equal between characters or words	between characters or words affected	
Close up normal interline spacing	each side of column linking lines	
Insert space between lines or paragraphs	or	
Reduce space between lines or paragraphs	or	
Reduce space between characters	between characters affected	
Reduce space between words	between words affected	

Appendix C:
Sample book contract

MEMORANDUM OF AGREEMENT

made this
BETWEEN

[hereinafter called 'the Author'] of the one part and
[hereinafter called 'the Publisher'] of the other part

WHEREBY IT IS AGREED between the parties hereto for themselves, their respective executors, administrators, and assigns [or successors as the case may be] as follows:

1. THE WORK

The Author shall prepare for publication to the approval of the Publisher a book tentatively titled

[hereinafter called 'the Work']

2. RIGHTS GRANTED

The Author hereby grants to the Publisher the sole and exclusive right and licence to produce and publish and further to licence the production and publication of the Work or any adaptation or any abridgement of the Work or any substantial part of the Work in all languages for the legal term of copyright throughout the world, in consideration of the payments hereinafter mentioned and subject to the terms and conditions hereinafter mentioned, but the Copyright in the Work shall remain vested in the Author.

3. DELIVERY OF THE WORK

The Author shall deliver to the Publisher not later than the day of..................... a double-spaced typescript of the Work suitable for use as compositor's copy, plus a duplicate, to make approximately 110 to 122 printed pages of a page size 216 times 138 millimetres, calculated at 450 words per page but with due allowance for illustrations and/or formulae.

4. STATE OF TYPESCRIPT

The typescript shall conform in style and appearance to the specification previously agreed with the Publisher. The Author shall include a Preface and Table of Contents, and, when proofs become available, Index, or hereby authorizes the Publisher to arrange for its compilation at the Author's expense.

5. ILLUSTRATIONS

The Author shall on delivery of the typescript supply to the Publisher without additional remuneration the necessary photographs, diagrams, or other materials from which to illustrate the Work in a state ready for reproduction. Diagrams may be supplied as rough sketches, to be transformed into artwork by the publisher's artists and at the Publisher's expense.

6. PERMISSIONS

The Author shall deliver with the typescript written permissions, with any permission fees paid by the Author, for publication in all editions of the Work of any graphic or textual material from published or unpublished work of others. If the Author does not obtain permissions, the Publisher is authorized to acquire them and to charge any permissions fees to the Author.

7. EDITING THE TYPESCRIPT

The Publisher shall be entitled to edit the typescript in accordance with its standard style of capitalization, punctuation, spelling and usage.

8. CORRECTIONS IN PROOF

The Author undertakes to read and correct the proofs of the Work and return the proofs promptly in accordance with the schedule notified by the Publisher. If the cost of Author's alterations to the proofs, excluding corrections of compositor's errors, exceeds ten per cent of the cost of composition, the excess costs shall be deductible from amounts due to the Author.

9. PUBLISHER'S UNDERTAKING

a] The Publisher shall publish the Work within a reasonable period of the acceptance of the final revised and satisfactory typescript such term including if appropriate illustrative matter and permissions as referred to in Clauses 5 and 6 above.

b] The Publisher shall have sole control of all details of design production, advertising, price, sale and terms of sale of the Work.

c] If the Publisher does not publish the Work within a reasonable period, the Author may then serve a written demand upon the Publisher to publish the Work within six months after receipt by the Publisher of the notice, and if the Publisher fails to comply with the Author's demand within the period provided, this Agreement shall terminate and all rights in the Work shall revert to the Author without further obligation or liability on the part of the Publisher.

10. AUTHOR'S WARRANTY

The Author hereby warrants to the Publisher that the Author has full power to make this Agreement, is the owner of the rights herein granted, that the Work is original to the Author and has not previously been published in any form in the territories covered by the Agreement nor is a violation or infringement of any existing copyright or licence, contains nothing defamatory and libellous, and does not contain any statements purporting to be facts that are untrue.

11. WARNINGS IN THE TEXT

The Author shall include in the text of the Work appropriate warnings concerning any particular hazards that may be involved in carrying out experiments or procedures described in the Work or involved in instructions, materials, or formulas in the Work, and shall explicitly mention relevant safety precautions, and give, if any accepted code of practice is followed, a reference to the relevant standard or code.

12. LIABILITY FOR AUTHOR'S PROPERTY

It is hereby declared that the Publisher is not an insurer of manuscripts, typescripts, photographs, drawings or other material delivered to the Publisher by or on behalf of the Author and will not in any circumstances be liable therefor.

13. COMPETING WORKS

The Author undertakes during the continuance of the Agreement not to prepare without the written consent of the Publisher any work likely to affect prejudicially the sales of the Work.

14. MORAL RIGHTS OF AUTHOR

The Author hereby asserts to the Publisher the Author's moral rights of paternity and integrity in the Work defined as follows:

a] the right of paternity shall mean the right of the Author to be identified by the Publisher as the author of the Work on or in each copy published and sold.

b] The right of integrity shall mean the right of the Author to object to the Publisher in the event of any derogatory treatment of the work by the Publisher to an extent which amounts to distortion or mutilation or which could be construed as otherwise prejudicial to the honour or reputation of the Author.

15. ROYALTIES

a] The Publisher shall pay to the Author a royalty of per cent of the net income received by the Publisher from the sale of the work in volume, sheet form or electronic form throughout the world.

b] No royalty shall be paid on copies presented to the Author or furnished for review, publicity, promotion, sample or similar purposes or destroyed or damaged by fire, water or any other cause, or returned for credit or refund to the Publisher.

c] Any increases in royalty rate provided in paragraph 15 [a] based upon the number of copies of the Work sold shall be separately computed for and applied to each edition of the Work.

d] No royalty shall be paid on copies sold by the Publisher at or below unit costs.

16. SUBSIDIARY RIGHTS

The Publisher shall have the exclusive right to sell or lease all subsidiary rights in the Work or any revised edition thereof including but not limited to translation rights, reproduction rights, electronic rights and quotation rights, and all income from such sale shall be divided equally between the publisher and the Author. The Author shall refer to the Publisher any enquiries received by the Author which relate to the exploitation of subsidiary rights in the Work.

17. ACCOUNTS

The Publisher shall render accounts of the sales of the Work as to December 31st of each year and all money due to the Author shall be paid to the Author by the succeeding April 1st provided, however, that no accounts need be rendered unless specifically demanded nor payment made in respect of any period in which the sum due is less than twenty five pounds, in which case the amount will be carried forward to the next accounting date, except where the book has been declared out of print by the Publisher or the Agreement has been terminated under the terms of Clause 22.

18. EXAMINATION OF ACCOUNTS

The Author or the authorized representatives of the Author shall have the right, upon written request, to examine the books of account of the Publisher, insofar as they relate to the sales of the Work, which examination shall be at the cost of the Author unless errors exceeding twenty five pounds shall be found to the disadvantage of the Author, in which case the cost shall be borne by the Publisher.

19. PRESENTATION COPIES

The Publisher shall present to each author after publication complimentary copies of the Work. Each author shall have the right to purchase further copies of the Work, and other books on the list of the Publisher, for personal use and not for resale at a discount of 25%.

20. NEW EDITIONS

a] The Author agrees to revise the Work when the Publisher deems it necessary. Except as provided below, the terms of this Agreement will apply to the revised Work.
b] If the Author is unable or unwilling for any reason to deliver a revised manuscript, acceptable to the Publisher and within the reasonable schedule requirement of the Publisher, the Publisher may have the revision prepared or completed by others and may charge the compensation payable to the revisers against the sums due to the Author or the estate of the Author in respect of the revised Work.
c] The Publisher shall have the right to use the Author's name in connection with the first and subsequent revisions, provided that the revisers are identified in the Work.

21. JOINT AUTHORSHIP

All persons executing this Agreement as the Author shall share in the expenses and benefits under this Agreement in the same proportion as their share in the royalties and proceeds, and shall be jointly and severally responsible for the obligations of the Author. In absence of a written agreement to the contrary, the Publisher may assume that each author is entitled to an equal share of all sums due and payable under this Agreement. The authors will furnish the Publisher with the agreed order of authorship credit, and if the authors do not agree, the Publisher shall determine the order.

22. TERMINATION

This Agreement shall automatically be terminated and all rights granted by the Author to the Publisher shall revert to the Author without prejudice to any claim which either party hereto may have against the other for money due and/or damages, if:

a] The Publisher fails to fulfil any of the provisions of this agreement within three months after written notification from the author of such failure.

b] An order is made for the liquidation of the Publisher other than for voluntary liquidation for the purpose of amalgamation or reconstruction only.

c] After the work is out of stock or out of print in all editions, the publisher has not within nine months of a written request of the Author issued a new edition or impression. After termination, any sums owing to the Author under the terms and Clauses 15 and 16 shall be paid to the Author.

23. NOTICE

Any notice or request under this Agreement shall be sufficiently given or made by posting the same in a registered letter addressed in the case of the publisher to the Managing Director at the current main address of the Publisher or in the other to the Author at the latest address held by the Publisher.

24. ARBITRATION

This Agreement shall be subject to, construed and interpreted according to the Law of England and any dispute or difference between the parties hereto which cannot be otherwise resolved shall be subject to the jurisidiction of the English courts in accordance with and subject to the provisions of the Arbitration Act 1950 or any statutory modification or re-enactment thereof for the time being in force.

25. ADVANCE (ON ROYALTIES)

The publisher's agree to pay the author on receipt and approval of the final manuscript.

IN WITNESS WHEREOF, the parties hereto have executed this Agreement on the date first above set forth.

SIGNED by the said Author

in the presence of

SIGNED on behalf of the Publisher by

in the presence of

Appendix D:
Guidelines for non-sexist language

American Psychological Association (1983) *Publication Manual*, (3rd edn).

Washington, DC: Author.

GUIDELINES FOR NONSEXIST LANGUAGE IN APA JOURNALS

Consideration of the Reader

Help the reader focus on the content of your paper by avoiding language that may cause irritation, flights of thought, or even momentary interruptions. Such sources of distraction include linguistic devices and constructions that might imply sexual, ethnic, or other kinds of bias.

Devices that attract attention to words, sounds, or other embellishments instead of to ideas are inappropriate in scientific writing. Avoid heavy alliteration, accidental rhyming, poetic expressions, and clichés. Use metaphors sparingly: although they can help simplify complicated ideas, metaphors can be distracting. *Avoid mixed metaphors* (e.g. *a theory representing one branch of a growing body of evidence*) and words with surplus or unintended meaning (e.g. *cop* for *police officer*), which may distract if not actually mislead the reader. Use figurative expressions with restraint and colorful expressions with care: these expressions can sound strained or forced.

APA as a publisher accepts journal authors' word choices unless those choices are inaccurate, unclear, or ungrammatical. Because APA as an organization is committed both to science and to the fair treatment of individuals and groups, however, authors of journal articles are required to avoid writing in a manner that reinforces questionable attitudes and assumptions about people.

2.12 *Guidelines for Nonsexist Language in APA Journals*

Language that reinforces sexism can spring from subtle errors in research design, inaccurate interpretation, or imprecise word choices. An investigator may unintentionally introduce bias into the research design, for example, by using stimulus materials and measures that suggest to one sex or the other what responses are 'appropriate'. Or, in interpretation, an investigator may make unwarranted generalizations about both men and women from data about one sex. Imprecise word choices, which occur frequently in journal writing, may be interpreted as biased, discriminatory, or demeaning even if they are not intended to be.

Advice on research design and interpretation is beyond the scope of the APA *Publication Manual*. However, in the spirit of the discussion on writing style in this chapter, the *Manual* does contain guidelines on nonsexist language to help authors recognize and change instances in which word choices may be inaccurate, misleading, or discriminatory (see Table 1).

In 1977 the APA adopted guidelines for nonsexist language, which appeared as Change Sheet 2 for the 1974 edition of the *Manual*. In 1982 the APA Publications and Communications Board adopted a policy that requires authors who are submitting their manuscripts to an APA journal to use nonsexist language, that is, to avoid in their manuscripts language that could be construed as sexist. The guidelines on nonsexist language adopted in 1977 are reproduced in Table 1 with minor editorial improvements and updating.

Sexism in journal writing may be classified into two categories: problems of designation and problems of evaluation.

Problems of designation. When you refer to a person or persons, choose words that are accurate, clear, and free from bias. Long-established cultural practice can exert a powerful, insidious, influence over even the most conscientious author. For example, the use of *man* as a generic noun can be ambiguous and may convey an implicit message that women are of secondary importance. You can choose nouns, pronouns, and adjectives to eliminate, or at least to minimize, the possibility of ambiguity in sex identity or sex role. In the examples in Table 1, problems of designation are divided into two subcategories: *ambiguity of referent*, when it is unclear whether the author means one sex or both sexes, and *stereotyping*, when the writing conveys unsupported or biased connotations about sex roles and identity.

Problems of evaluation.   Scientific writing, as an extension of science, should be free of implied or irrelevant evaluation of the sexes. Difficulties may derive from the habitual use of clichés or familiar expressions, such as 'man and wife.' The use of *man and wife* together implies differences in the freedom and activities of each and may inappropriately prompt the reader to evaluate the roles. Thus, *husband* and *wife* are parallel, and *man* and *woman* are parallel, but *man* and *wife* are not. In the examples in Table 1, problems of evaluation, like problems of designation, are divided into *ambiguity of referent* and *stereotyping*.

Avoiding sexist language.   The task of changing language may seem awkward at first. Nevertheless, careful attention to meaning and practice in rephrasing will overcome any initial difficulty. The result of such effort, and the purpose of the Table 1 guidelines, is accurate, unbiased communication.

2.13 *Avoiding Ethnic Bias*

Like language that may be interpreted as sexist, language that may be construed as ethnically biased can be classified into problems of designation and problems of evaluation.

Problems of designation.   Styles and preferences for nouns referring to ethnic groups change over time. In some cases, even members of a group disagree about the preferred name at a specific time. You should try to ascertain the most acceptable current terms and use them. Consideration for your audience should prevail.

Problems of evaluation.   The majority of instances of implied irrelevant evaluation seem to occur when the writer uses one group (usually the writer's *own* group) as the standard against which others are assessed. Unfortunately, the basis for negative comparisons is usually established during the planning of the research, for example, by the choice of empirical measures.

At the writing stage, avoid language that suggests evaluation. An example of implied evaluation is found in the term *culturally deprived* when it is used to describe a single group rather than to compare two or more groups. Using the term to describe one group of subjects – *without the supporting data required in scientific writing* – implies that one culture is a universally accepted standard against which others are judged. As a test of implied evaluation, substitute another group (e.g., your own) for the group being discussed. If you are offended by the revised statement, there is probably bias in the original statement.

Table 1 Guidelines for Nonsexist Language in APA
Journals

Examples of common usage	Alternatives
Problems of Designation: **Ambiguity of Referent**	
1. The *client* is usually the best judge of the value of *his* counseling.	The *client* is usually the best judge of the value of counseling. [Comment: *His* deleted] The client is usually the best judge of the value of his *or her* counseling [Comment: *Or her* added (Use sparingly to avoid monotonous repetition.)] *Clients* are usually the best judges of the value of the counseling *they* receive. [Comment: Changed to plural] The best judge of the value of counseling is usually *the client*. [Comment: Rephrased)]
2. *Man's search for* knowledge has led *him* into ways of learning that bear examination.	*The search* for knowledge has led *us* into ways of learning that bear examination. [Comment: Rephrased in first person] *People* have continually sought knowledge. The search has led *them* into ways of learning that bear examination. [Comment: Changed to plural and rewritten in two sentences]
3. man, mankind	people, humanity, human beings, humankind, human species
man's achievements	human achievements, achievements of the human species
the average man	the average person, people in general
man a project	staff a project, hire personnel, employ staff
man–machine interface	user–system interface, person-system interface, human-machine interface
manpower	work force, personnel, workers, human resources [Comment: Various terms substituted for each example]

4. The use of experiments in psychology presupposes the mechanistic nature of *man*

The use of experiments in psychology presupposes the mechanistic nature of the *human being.* [Comment: Noun substituted]

5. This interference phenomenon, called learned helplessness, has been, demonstrated in rats, cats, fish, dogs, monkeys, and *men.*

This interference phenomenon, learned helplessness, has been demonstrated in rats, cats, fish, dogs, monkeys, and *humans.* [Comment: Noun substituted]

6. Responsivity in the premature *infant* may be secondary to *his* heightened level of autonomic arousal.

Responsivity in the premature *infant* may be secondary to *the* heightened level of autonomic arousal. [Comment: *His* changed to *the*]

Responsivity in premature *infants* may be secondary to *their* heightened levels of autonomic arousal. [Comment: Rewritten in the plural]

7. First the *individual* becomes aroused by violations of *his* personal space, and then *he* attributes the cause of this arousal to other people in *his* environment.

First *we* become aroused by violations of *our* personal space, and then *we* attribute the cause of this arousal to other people in *the* environment. [Comment: First-person pronouns substituted for the noun and *he* and *his:* *his* changed to *the*]

First *one* becomes aroused by violations of personal space, and then *one* attributes the cause of this arousal to other people in *the* environment. [Comment: *One* substituted: *his* omitted or changed to *the*]

8. Much has been written about the effect that a *child's* position among *his* siblings has on *his* intellectual development.

Much has been written about the relationships between sibling position and intellectual development in *children*. [Comment: Rewritten: plural introduced]

9. Subjects were 16 girls and 16 boys. Each *child* was to place a car on *his* board so that two cars and boards looked alike

Each child was to place a car on *his* or *her* board so that two cars and boards looked alike. [Comment: *His* changed to *his* or *her* or to *her* or *his* (Use sparingly to avoid monotonous repetition.)]

10. Each person's alertness was measured by the difference between *his* obtained relaxation score and *his* obtained arousal score.

Each person's alertness was measured by the difference between *the* obtained relaxation and arousal scores. [Comment: *His* changed to *the*: plural introduced]

11. The client's husband *lets* her teach part-time

The client's husband "*lets*" her teach part-time.

The husband says he "*lets*" the client teach part-time

The client *says her husband "lets"* her teach part-time

[Comment: Punctuation added to clarify that the location of the bias is with the husband and wife, not with the author. If necessary, rewrite to clarify as allegation. (See Example 24.)]

Problems of Designation: Stereotyping

12. males, females

men, women, boys, girls, adults, children, adolescents [Comment: Specific nouns reduce possibility of stereotypic bias and often clarify discussion. Use *male* and *female* as adjectives where appropriate and relevant (female experimenter, male subject). Avoid unparallel usage such as 10 *men* and 16 *females*.]

13. Research scientists often neglect their *wives* and *children*.

Research scientists often neglect their *spouses* and *children*. [Comment: Alternative wording acknowledges that women as well as men are research scientists.]

14. When a *test developer* or *test user* fails to satisfy these requirements, *he* should . . .

When *test developers* or *test users* fail to satisfy these requirements, *they* should . . . [Comment: Same as Example 13]

15. the psychologist . . . *he*

    the therapist . . . *he*

    the nurse . . . *she*
    the teacher . . . *she*

psychologists . . . *they*: the psychologist . . . *she*

therapists . . . *they*: the therapist . . . *she* or *he*

nurses . . . *they*: nurse . . . *he*
teachers . . . *they*: teacher . . . *he*
[Comment: Be specific, change to plural if discussing women as well as men, or use *he or she*. Do not use *s/he*.]

16. woman doctor, lady lawyer, male nurse

doctor, physician, lawyer, nurse [Comment: Specify sex only if it is a variable or if sex designation is necessary to the discussion ("13 female doctors and 22 male

	doctors"). *Woman* and *lady* are nouns: *female* is the adjective counterpart to *male*.]
17. mothering	parenting, nurturing (or specify exact behaviour) [Comment: Noun substituted]
18. chairman (of an academic department)	Use *chairperson* or *chair*: use *chairman* only if it is known that the institution has established that form as an official title. [Comment: *Department head* may be appropriate: however, the term is not synonymous with *chair* and *chairperson* at all institutions.]
chairman (presiding officer of a committee or meeting)	chairperson, chair, moderator, discussion leader [Comment: In parliamentary usage, *chairman* is the official term and should not be changed. Alternatives are acceptable in most writing.]
19. Only *freshmen* were eligible for the project.	No alternative if academic standing is meant
All the students had matriculated for 3 years, but the majority were still *freshmen*.	No alternative if academic standing is meant
	[Comment: *First-year student* is often an acceptable alternative to *freshman*, but in these examples, *freshmen* is used for accuracy.]
20. foreman, policeman, mailman	supervisor or superintendent, police officer, postal worker or letter carrier [Comment: Noun substituted]

Problems of Evaluation: Ambiguity of Referent

21. The authors acknowledge the assistance of *Mrs John Smith*.	The authors acknowledge the assistance of *Jane Smith*. [Comment: Use given names.]
22. men and women, sons and daughters, boys and girls, husbands and wives	women and men, daughters and sons, girls and boys, wives and husbands [Comment: Vary the order if content does not require traditional order]

Problems of Evaluation: Stereotyping

23. men and girls	men and women, women and men, boys and girls [Comment: Use parallel terms. Of course, use *men* and *girls* if that is literally what is meant.]

24. The client's husband lets her teach part-time

The client teaches part-time. [Comment: The author of this example intended to communicate the working status of the woman but inadvertently revealed a stereotype about husband–wife relationships. (See Example 11.)]

25. ambitious men and aggressive women

ambitious women and men, ambitious people

aggressive men and women, aggressive people

cautious men and timid women

cautious women and men, cautious people

timid men and women, timid people

[Comment: Some adjectives, depending on whether the person described is a man or a woman, connote bias. The examples illustrate some common usages that may not always convey exact meaning, especially when paired, as in column 1.]

26. The boys chose typically male toys

The boys chose (specify).

The client's behavior was typically female.

The client's behavior was (specify). [Comment: Being specific reduces possibility of stereotypic bias.]

27. woman driver

driver [Comment: If specifying sex is necessary, avoid biased clichés. Use *female driver*, or write "The driver was a woman."]

28. The *girls* in the office greeted all clients.

receptionists, secretaries, office assistants [Comment: Noun substituted]

29. coed

student [Comment: Noun substituted. If specification of sex is necessary, use *female* student.]

30. women's lib, women's libber

women's movement, feminist, supporter of women's movement [Comment: Noun substituted]

31. Subjects were 16 men and 4 women. *The women were housewives*.

The men were (specify). and the women were (specify). [Comment: Women and men described in parallel terms or description of both omitted. Do not use *housewife* to identify occupation, a term that indicates sex and marital status and excludes men. Use *homemaker*, which includes men.]

References

Baker, J. (1987) *Copy Prep*, Blueprint, London.

Bennett, A. (1994) *Writing Home*, Faber & Faber, London.

Brande, D. (1934) *Becoming a Writer*, Harcourt Brace, New York.

Bradbury, R. (1990) *Zen in the Art of Writing: Essays on Creativity*, Joshua Odell editions, Capra Press, Santa Barbara, California.

Branscombe, M. (1991) The Data Protection Act: what you need to know. *PC Answers*, **1**(3), 56–7.

Bryman, A. (1988) *Quantity and Quality in Social Research*, Unwin Hyman, London.

Burnard, P. and Morrison, P. (1992) *Self Disclosure: A Contemporary Analysis*, Avebury, Aldershot.

— (1994) *Nursing Research in Action*, 2nd edn, Macmillan, London.

Butler, R. (1995) Forever English. *Independent on Sunday*, 12 February.

Canter, D. (1994) *Criminal Shadows*, HarperCollins, London.

Carey, G. V. (1976) *Mind the Stop*, Penguin, Harmondsworth.

Chapman & Hall, *Guide for Authors: Presentation of Illustrations*, Chapman & Hall, London.

Clairborne, R. (1990) *The Life and Times of the English Language: The History of our Marvellous Native Tongue*, Bloomsbury, London.

Classe, A. (1995) Portable peace of mind. *PC Direct*, January.

Docherty, T. (ed.) (1993) *Postmodernism: A Reader*, Harvester Wheatsheaf, New York.

The Economist Pocket Style Book (1986) The Economist Publications Ltd, London.

Eddings, J. (1994) *How the Internet Works*, Ziff Davis Press, Emeryville, California.

Edmunds, N. (1995) Suite success. *PC Direct*, January.

Fadiman, C. (1944) *Reading I've Liked*, Hamish Hamilton, London.

Field, P. A. and Morse, J. M. (1985) *Nursing Research: The Application of Qualitative Approaches*, Croom Helm, London.

Findlater, R. (ed). (1984) *Author! Author!*, Faber & Faber, London.

Gash, S. (1989) *Effective Literature Searching for Students*, Gower, Aldershot.

Giles, K. and Hedge, N. (1994) *The Manager's Good Study Guide*, Open University Press, Milton Keynes.

Gillett, H. (1990) *Study Skills: A Guide for Health Care Professionals*, Distance Learning Centre, South Bank Polytechnic, London.

Glaser, B. and Strauss, A. L. (1967) *The Discovery of Grounded Theory*, Aldine, New York.

Gowers, E. (1962) *The Complete Plain Words*, Penguin, Harmondsworth; 3rd edn (1986), HMSO.

Grimond, J. (1986) *The Economist Pocket Style Book*, The Economist, London.

Gunning, R. (1968) *The Technique of Clear Writing*, 2nd edn, McGraw-Hill, London.

Hahn, H. and Stout, R. (1994) *The Internet Yellow Pages*, Osborne McGraw-Hill, Berkeley, California.

Hansen, K. J. and Waterman, R. C. (1966) Evaluation of research in business education. *National Business Education Quarterly*, **35**, 81–4.

Harrison, N. (1985) *Writing English: A User's Manual*, Croom Helm, London.

Howard, K. and Sharp, J. A. (1983) *The Management of A Student Research Project:* Gower, Aldershot.

Hudson, K. (1978) *The Jargon of the Professions,* Macmillan, London.

Jourard, S. (1971) *Self-Disclosure: An Experimental Analysis of the Transparent Self,* Wiley, New York.

Kirkman, J. (1992) *Good Style: Writing for Science and Technology,* E and FN Spon, London.

Larson, M. (1986) *Literary Agents: How to Get and Work with the Right One for You,* Writer's Digest Books, Cincinnati, Ohio.

Lessing, D. (1984) Into the labyrinth. In R. Findlater (ed.), *Author! Author!,* Faber & Faber, London.

Levi, P. (1989) *Other People's Trades,* Abacus, London.

Levine, J. R. and Baroudi, C. (1993) *The Internet for Dummies,* IDG Books, San Mateo, California.

Maxwell, W. B. (1924) The sin of silence. In R. Findlater (ed.), *Author! Author!,* Faber & Faber, London.

Orem, D. (1980) *Nursing: Concepts of Practice,* 2nd edn., McGraw-Hill, New York.

Polit, D. F. and Hungler, B. P. (1991) *Nursing Research: Principles and Methods,* 4th edn, Lippincott, Philadelphia.

Que Corporation (1984) *The Internet Resource: Quick Reference,* Que, Indianapolis.

Scott Fitzgerald, F. (1985) Afternoon of an author. In L. W. Phillips (ed.), *F. Scott Fitzgerald on Writing,* Scribner, New York.

Somer, B. and Somer, R. (1991) *A Practical Guide to Behavioural Research: Tools and Techniques,* 3rd edn, Oxford University Press, New York.

Strong, W. (1991) *Writing Incisively: Do-it-yourself Prose Surgery,* McGraw-Hill, New York.

Strunk, W. and White, E. B. (1979) *The Elements of Style,* Macmillan, New York.

Turk, C. and Kirkman, E. B. (1989) *Effective Writing: Improving Scientific, Technical and Business Communication,* 2nd edn, E and FN Spon, London.

Turner, B. (ed.) (1992) *The Writer's Handbook,* Macmillan/PEN, London

Wells, G. (1981) *The Successful Author's Handbook,* Macmillan, Basingstoke.

Wittgenstein, L. (1922; 1961) *Tractatus Logico-Philosophicus,* Routledge & Kegan Paul, London.

Wodehouse, P. G. (1934) *Thank you Jeeves.* In P. G. Wodehouse, *The Jeeves Omnibus,* Hutchinson, London.

Wright Mills, C. (1959) *The Sociological Imagination,* Penguin; Oxford University Press, Oxford.

Further reading

Adams, J. (1984) *How to Sell What You Write*, Putnams, New York.

Adler, W. (1982) *Inside Publishing*, Bobbs-Merrill, New York.

American Society of Authors (1983) *The Complete Guide to Writing Non-Fiction*, Writers Digest Books, Cincinnati, Ohio.

Applin, L. (1993) Report writing for managers. *Senior Nurse*, **13**(3), 7–8.

Balfe, A. (1989) *Master Your Hard Disk*, Sigma, Wilmslow

Ball, M. J. and Hannah, K. J. (1984) *Using Computers in Nursing*, Reston Publishing, Reston, V.A.

Barlow, G. (1978) *Typesetting and Composition*, Blueprint, London

Belkin, G. S. (1984) *Getting Published: A Guide for Business People and Other Professionals*, Wiley, New York.

Berger, R. M. (1991) Four steps to getting your paper published. *Child and Youth Care Forum*, **20**, 211–14.

Burnard, P. (1990) So you think you need a computer? *The Professional Nurse*, **6**(2), 119–20.

— (1994) *Personal Computing Skills for Health Professionals*, Chapman & Hall, London.

— (1995) *Health Care Computing*, Chapman & Hall, London.

Butcher, J. (1981) *Copy Editing: The Cambridge Handbook*, Cambridge University Press, Cambridge.

Corwin, J. (1984) *How to Become a Bestselling Author*, Writer's Digest Books, Cincinnati, Ohio.

Crouchner, P. (1989) *Communications and Networks: A Handbook for the First Time User,* Sigma, Wilmslow.

Day, R. (1988) *How to Write and Publish a Scientific Paper*, 3rd edn, ISI Press, Philadelphia.

de Presno, O. (1989) *The Shareware Handbook*, Sigma, Wilmslow.

Dies, R. R. (1993) Writing for publication: overcoming common obstacles. *International Journal of Group Psychotherapy*, **43**(2), 243–9.

Dynes, R. (1989) Using creative writing. *British Journal of Occupational Therapy*, **52**, 151–2.

Englert, C. S. (1992) Writing instruction from a sociocultural perspective: the holistic, dialogic, and social enterprise of writing. *Journal of Learning Disabilities*, **25**, 153–77.

Evans, H, Evans, M. and Nelki, A. (1979) *The Picture Researcher's Handbook*, David & Charles, London.

Evans, H. (1986) *Editing and Design: A Five Volume Manual of English Typography and Layout: 1. Newsman's English; 2. Handling Newspaper Text; 3. News Headlines; 4. Pictures on a Page; 5. Newspaper Design*, Heinemann, for the National Council for the Training of Journalists, London.

Evesham, D. A. (1989) *Developing Real Time Systems*, Sigma, Wilmslow.

Ewbank, K. and Gee, S. M. (1989) *Quattro Quickstep*, Sigma, Wilmslow.

Fuchs, L. S. and Fuchs, D. (1993) Writing research reports for publication: recommendations for new authors. *Remedial and Special Education (RASE)*, **14**(3), 39–46.

Goldin, S. and Sky, K. (1982) The Business of Being a Writer: Harper & Row, New York.

Goldstein, H. (1993) Writing to be read: the place of the essay in social work literature. *Families in Society*, **74**(7), 441–6.

Graham, S., Schwartz, S. S., MacArthur, C. A. (1993) Knowledge of writing and the composing process, attitude toward writing, and self-efficacy for students with and without learning disabilities. *Journal of Learning Disabilities*, **26**(4), 237–49.

Greenfield, H. (1986) *Books: From Writer to Reader*, Crown, New York.

Gregg, N. and Hoy, C. (1990) Referencing: the cohesive use of pronouns in the written narrative of college underprepared writers, nondisabled writers, and writers with learning disabilities. *Journal of Learning Disabilities*, **23**, 57–63.

Grimond, J. (1986) *The Economist Pocket Style Book*, The Economist, London.

Gross, G. (1985) *Editors on Editing: An Inside View of what Editors Really Do*, Harper & Row, New York.

Harrison, N. (1985) *Writing English: A User's Manual*, Croom Helm, London.

Heenan, A. (1993) Get it write. *Nursing Times*, **89**(7), 24–5.

Hollins, T. (1989) *WordStar: The Ultimate Guide*, Sigma, Wilmslow.

Houp, K. W. and Pearsall, T. E. (1988) *Reporting Technical Information*, 6th edn, Macmillan, New York.

Kamali, A. (1991) Writing a sociological student term paper: steps and scheduling. *Teaching Sociology*, **19**, 506–9.

Karach, A. and Roach, D. (1992) Collaborative writing, consciousness raising, and practical feminist ethics. *Women's Studies International Forum*, **15**(2), 303–8.

Kitson, G.C. (1993) On writing: getting started, getting stuck, and getting finished. *Marriage and Family Review*, **18**(1/2), 143–59.

Koch, R. and Rankin, J. (eds) (1987) *Computers and Their Application in Nursing*, Harper & Row, London.

Lewis, M. (1987) *Writing to Win*, McGraw-Hill, London.

— (1989) *Inside Dbase*, Sigma, Wilmslow.

Maclure, M. (1994) Language and discourse: the embrace of uncertainty: review essay. *British Journal of Sociology of Education*, **15**(2), 283–300.

Martin, J. (1992) Scholarship and professionalism: a personal narrative. *Journal of Counseling and Development*, **70**, 563–4.

Mayer, D. (1983) *Literary Agents: A Writer's Guide*: Pushcart Press, New York.

McKenzie, A. (1992) So, you want to be a writer? *Police Review*, **100**, 1414–15.

McKeown, S. (1992) Microcomputer software: programs for writing and spelling. *British Journal of Special Education*, **19**, 100.

McLoughlin, D. (1992) Use of creative writing in palliative care. *Reading Therapy Newsletter*, **4**(3), 5–14.

Mumby, F. A. and Norrie, I. (1974) *Publishing and Bookselling*, 5th edn, Cape, London.

O'Connor, M. and Woodford, F. P. (1978) *Writing Scientific Papers in English*, Pitman, Oxford.

Parahoo, K. and Reid, N. (1988) Research skills no. 3: writing a research proposal. *Nursing Times*, **84**, 49–52.

Parahoo, K. and Reid, N. (1988) Research skills no. 4: writing up a research report. *Nursing Times*, **84**, 63–7.

Parry, A. (1993) How to ... write an abstract or summary. *Physiotherapy*, **79**(7), 472–3.

Peacock, J., Berrill, C. and Barnard, M. (1986) *The Print and Production Manual*, Blueprint, London.

Petersen, C. (1970) *The Bantam Story: Thirty Years of Paperback Publishing*, Bantam Books, New York.

Peterson, F. and Kesselman-Truket (1982) *The Author's Handbook*, Prentice Hall, Englewood Cliffs.

Pollard, N. (1993) On doing the write thing. *Reading Therapy Newsletter*, **5**(2), 7–9.

Rankin, J. L., Bruning, R. H., Timme, V. L., Katkanant, C. (1993) Is writing affected by spelling performance and beliefs about spelling? *Applied Cognitive Psychology*, **7**(2), 155–69.

Roberts, K. A. (1993) Toward a sociology of writing. *Teaching Sociology*, **21**(4), 317–24.

Rosnow, R. L. and Rosnow, M. (1986) *Writing Papers in Psychology: A Student Guide*, Wadsworth, Belmont, California.

Salomone, P. R. (1993) Trade secrets for crafting a conceptual article. *Journal of Counseling and Development*, **72**(1), 73–6.

Seligman, S. and Kelly, C. (1990) Writing and publishing books in counseling: a survey of authors. *Journal of Counseling and Development*, **69**, 42–5.

Smith, C. (1989) *The PC Upgrade Handbook*, Sigma, Wilmslow.

Spooner, F. (1993) Writing for publication in journals for practitioners: suggestions for teachers and early career researchers. *Remedial and Special Education (RASE)*, **14**(3), 47–52.

Strunk, W. and White, E. B. (1979) *The Elements of Style: Macmillan*, New York.

Sweeney, M. A. (1985) *The Nurse's Guide to Computers*, Macmillan, New York.

Turk, C. and Kirkman, J. (1989) *Effective Writing: Improving Scientific, Technical and Business Communication*, 2nd edn, E. and F.N. Spon, London.

Walker, D. (1985) Writing and reflection. In D. Boud, R. Keogh and D. Walker (eds), *Reflection: Turning Experience into Learning*, Kogan Page, London.

Weitz, R. (1991) Teaching writing for publication. *Teaching Sociology*, **19**, 414–17.

Woodhead, N. (1990) *Hypertext and HyperCard – Theory and Applications*, Sigma, Wilmslow.

Zeisel, H. (1985) *Say It With Figures*, revised edn, Harper & Row, New York.

Index